MILITARY AND VETERAN ISSUES

IMPROVEMENTS NEEDED IN THE VA HEALTH CARE SYSTEM

Military and Veteran Issues

Additional books and e-books in this series can be found on Nova's website under the Series tab.

Health Care in Transition

Additional books and e-books in this series can be found on Nova's website under the Series tab.

MILITARY AND VETERAN ISSUES

IMPROVEMENTS NEEDED IN THE VA HEALTH CARE SYSTEM

CHARLES COPELAND
EDITOR

snova
New York

Library of Congress Cataloging-in-Publication Data

ISBN: 978-1-53615-971-4

Published by Nova Science Publishers, Inc. † New York

CONTENTS

PREFACE

Nearly 40,000 providers hold privileges in VHA's 170 VA Medical Centers (VAMCs). VAMCs must identify and review any concerns that arise about the clinical care their providers deliver.

Chapter 1 examines, among other things, selected VAMCs' reviews of providers' clinical care after concerns are raised and VHA's oversight of these reviews, and VAMCs' reporting of providers to the NPDB and SLBs and VHA's oversight of reporting.

Chapter 2 summarizes the implementation and oversight of VHA processes for reviewing and reporting providers after quality and safety concerns have been raised at selected VA medical centers.

Veterans suffer a disproportionately higher rate of suicide than the civilian population. Chapter 3 focuses on the extent to which VHA conducts activities for its suicide prevention media outreach campaign, and evaluates the effectiveness of its campaign. The Faster Care for Veterans Act of 2016 called for the Department of Veterans Affairs (VA) to conduct a pilot program under which veterans can use an Internet website or mobile application to schedule and confirm appointments at the department's medical facilities.

Chapter 4 examines the extent to which VHA (conducts activities for its suicide prevention media outreach campaign, and evaluates the effectiveness of its campaign.

VAMCs use reusable medical equipment (RME) which must be reprocessed—that is, cleaned, disinfected, or sterilized—between uses. Improper reprocessing of RME can negatively affect patient care. To help ensure the safety of veterans, VHA policy establishes requirements VAMCs must follow when reprocessing RME and requires a number of related oversight efforts. Chapters 5 and 6 discuss VHA's oversight of VAMCs' adherence to RME policies and challenges VAMCs face in operating their Sterile Processing Services programs, and any efforts by VHA to address these challenges.

VHA has designated patient advocates at each VAMC to receive and document feedback from veterans or their representatives, including requests for information, compliments, and complaints. Chapter 7 examines the extent to which VHA has provided guidance on the governance of the program; provided guidance on staffing the program; assessed the training needs of patient advocates and monitored training completion; and monitored patient advocacy program data-entry practices and reviewed program data.

Community-based outpatient clinics (CBOC) are an important part of the Department of Veterans Affairs' (VA) Veterans Health Administration (VHA) health care delivery system. These clinics are geographically separate from VA medical centers (VAMC) and provide outpatient services, including primary care and mental health care. Chapter 8 reviews VHA's use of contracts to carry out core functions.

Selected Department of Veterans Affairs' (VA) medical centers (VAMC) use generally similar approaches for managing their pharmacy inventories. Chapter 9 describes approaches selected VAMCs use to manage their pharmacy inventories and assesses the extent to which VA oversees VAMCs' efforts to manage their pharmacy inventories.

The Veterans Health Administration (VHA) has made progress improving opioid safety through its Opioid Safety Initiative (OSI). Chapter 10 examines the extent to which VHA has met OSI goals established in 2014 and (2) the extent to which VHA providers adhere to key opioid risk mitigation strategies.

In: Improvements Needed in the VA … ISBN: 978-1-53615-971-4
Editor: Charles Copeland

Chapter 1

IMPROVED POLICIES AND OVERSIGHT NEEDED FOR REVIEWING AND REPORTING PROVIDERS FOR QUALITY AND SAFETY CONCERNS*

United States Government Accountability Office

ABBREVIATIONS

FPPE	focused professional practice evaluation
NPDB	National Practitioner Data Bank
SLB	state licensing board
VA	Department of Veterans Affairs
VAMC	Department of Veterans Affairs medical center
VHA	Veterans Health Administration
VISN	Veterans Integrated Service Network August 3, 2018

* This is an edited, reformatted and augmented version of United States Government Accountability Office; Report to Congressional Requesters, Publication No. GAO-18-63, dated November 2017.

WHY GAO DID THIS STUDY

Nearly 40,000 providers hold privileges in VHA's 170 VAMCs. VAMCs must identify and review any concerns that arise about the clinical care their providers deliver. Depending on the findings from the review, VAMC officials may take an adverse privileging action against a provider that either limits the care a provider is allowed to deliver at the VAMC or prevents the provider from delivering care altogether.

GAO was asked to review VHA processes for reviewing concerns about providers' clinical care. This chapter examines, among other things, selected VAMCs' (1) reviews of providers' clinical care after concerns are raised and VHA's oversight of these reviews, and (2) VAMCs' reporting of providers to the NPDB and SLBs and VHA's oversight of reporting. GAO visited a non-generalizable selection of five VAMCs selected for the complexity of services offered and variation in location. GAO reviewed VHA policies and files from the five selected VAMCs, and interviewed VHA, VISN, and VAMC officials. GAO also evaluated VHA's practices using federal internal control standards.

WHAT GAO RECOMMENDS

GAO is making four recommendations, including for VA to direct VHA to require VAMCs to document reviews of providers' clinical care after concerns are raised, develop timeliness requirements for these reviews, and ensure proper VISN oversight of such reviews as well as timely VAMC reporting of providers to the NPDB and SLBs. VA concurred with GAO's recommendations and described steps it will take to implement them.

WHAT GAO FOUND

Department of Veterans Affairs (VA) medical center (VAMC) officials are responsible for reviewing the clinical care delivered by their privileged providers—physicians and dentists who are approved to independently perform specific services—after concerns are raised. The five VAMCs GAO selected for review collectively required review of 148 providers from October 2013 through March 2017 after concerns were raised about their clinical care. GAO found that these reviews were not always documented or conducted in a timely manner. GAO identified these providers by reviewing meeting minutes from the committee responsible for requiring these types of reviews at the respective VAMCs, and through interviews with VAMC officials. The selected VAMCs were unable to provide documentation of these reviews for almost half of the 148 providers. Additionally, the VAMCs did not start the reviews of 16 providers for 3 months to multiple years after the concerns were identified. GAO found that VHA policies do not require documentation of all types of clinical care reviews and do not establish timeliness requirements. GAO also found that the Veterans Health Administration (VHA) does not adequately oversee these reviews at VAMCs through its Veterans Integrated Service Networks (VISN), which are responsible for overseeing the VAMCs. Without documentation and timely reviews of providers' clinical care, VAMC officials may lack information needed to reasonably ensure that VA providers are competent to provide safe, high quality care to veterans and to make appropriate decisions about these providers' privileges.

GAO also found that from October 2013 through March 2017, the five selected VAMCs did not report most of the providers who should have been reported to the National Practitioner Data Bank (NPDB) or state licensing boards (SLB) in accordance with VHA policy. The NPDB is an electronic repository for critical information about the professional conduct and competence of providers. GAO found that

- selected VAMCs did not report to the NPDB eight of nine providers who had adverse privileging actions taken against them or who resigned during an investigation related to professional competence or conduct, as required by VHA policy, and
- none of these nine providers had been reported to SLBs.

GAO found that officials at the selected VAMCs misinterpreted or were not aware of VHA policies and guidance related to NPDB and SLB reporting processes resulting in providers not being reported. GAO also found that VHA and the VISNs do not conduct adequate oversight of NPDB and SLB reporting practices and cannot reasonably ensure appropriate reporting of providers. As a result, VHA's ability to provide safe, high quality care to veterans is hindered because other VAMCs, as well as non-VA health care entities, will be unaware of serious concerns raised about a provider's care. For example, GAO found that after one VAMC failed to report to the NPDB or SLBs a provider who resigned to avoid an adverse privileging action, a non-VA hospital in the same city took an adverse privileging action against that same provider for the same reason 2 years later.

November 15, 2017

The Honorable David P. Roe
Chairman
Committee on Veterans' Affairs
House of Representatives

Dear Mr. Chairman:

The Department of Veterans Affairs' (VA) Veterans Health Administration (VHA) operates one of the largest health care systems in the nation, and nearly 40,000 providers hold privileges at its 170 VA medical centers (VAMC).[1] As in all health care delivery settings, VAMCs are responsible for ensuring that their providers deliver safe care to patients. If a concern about a provider's clinical care arises at any point, it is the VAMC's responsibility to review the provider's clinical care.[2]

---

[1] Privileges are the specific set of clinical services that a provider is approved to perform independently at a medical facility, based on an assessment of the provider's professional performance, judgement, clinical competence, and skills. For the purposes of this report, we use the term "provider" to refer to physicians and dentists.

[2] Examples of concerns about a provider's clinical care range from a provider not adequately documenting information about a patient visit to a provider practicing in a manner that is

Depending on the nature of the concern and the findings from their review, VAMC leadership officials may take adverse privileging actions against providers that either limit the care they are allowed to deliver at the facility or prevent the providers from delivering care altogether. VAMC officials are also required to report the providers they take adverse privileging actions against to the National Practitioner Data Bank (NPDB), which is used by other VAMCs, non-VA hospitals, and other health care entities to obtain information on providers with a history of substandard care and misconduct.[3] VAMC officials are also required to report providers to state licensing boards (SLB) when there are serious concerns about a provider's clinical practice. The SLB can then investigate and determine if the provider's license to practice medicine should be suspended, restricted, or revoked.

Congress and VA have taken recent steps to make the adverse privileging action process more efficient and more transparent. For example, the Department of Veterans Affairs Accountability and Whistleblower Protection Act of 2017 shortens the appeals process timeframe when a VAMC proposes taking an adverse privileging action.[4] While these actions may shorten the time period for reviewing and rendering a decision on taking an adverse privileging action, questions remain about the extent to which VAMC leadership officials review providers' clinical care after concerns are raised and, when appropriate, take adverse privileging actions against these providers and report them to the NPDB or SLBs. For example, there have been recent whistleblower complaints from VAMC providers to the U.S. Office of Special Counsel

unsafe or inconsistent with industry standards of care. Such concerns may arise, for example, as part of VAMCs' routine performance monitoring or from patient complaints.

3 The NPDB is an electronic repository administered by the U.S. Department of Health and Human Services that collects and releases information on providers who either have been disciplined by a state licensing board, professional society, or health care entity, such as a hospital, or have been named in a medical malpractice settlement or judgment. Industry standards call for health care entities to query the NPDB and verify with the appropriate state licensing board that a provider's medical licenses are current and in good standing before appointing a provider to the entity's medical staff and when renewing clinical privileges.

4 Pub. L. No. 115-41, § 208, 131 Stat. 862, 878 (2017), codified, as amended, at 38 U.S.C. § 7462.

alleging that VAMC leadership officials have not adequately reviewed and addressed issues regarding providers' clinical care after concerns have been raised.[5] According to the whistleblowers, specific providers have delivered care in a manner that is unsafe and inconsistent with industry standards of care, such as performing unnecessary procedures on veterans, without adequate reviews and actions taken by VAMC leadership.

Questions have also been raised about the extent to which VHA gives performance pay—a component of VA provider compensation—to providers who have had an adverse privileging action taken against them. Performance pay is an annual lump sum payment given to providers based on the extent to which the provider achieves specific goals in a given fiscal year. In July 2013, we reported that providers who were the subject of adverse actions, including adverse privileging actions, received performance pay for the same year the actions were taken.[6]

You asked us to review the processes VHA has in place to review providers' clinical care after concerns arise and the extent to which providers receive performance pay when concerns are confirmed. In this chapter, we examine

1. VAMCs' reviews of providers' clinical care after concerns are raised and VHA's oversight of these reviews;
2. VAMCs' reporting of providers to the NPDB and SLBs and VHA's oversight of these processes; and
3. the extent to which VAMCs give performance pay to providers who have had an adverse privileging action taken against them.

---

[5] The Office of Special Counsel is charged with protecting federal employees from prohibited personnel practices, such as retaliation against whistleblowing, discrimination, and nepotism. The Office of Special Counsel also handles other claims of wrongdoing from current employees, former employees, and applicants for federal employment including wrongdoing that presents a substantial and specific danger to public health or safety.

[6] Our 2013 report focused on disciplinary and adverse actions beyond adverse privileging actions, such as letters of reprimand and suspension without pay. One of the five providers identified in the 2013 report had been the subject of an adverse privileging action; the other four providers had other types of actions taken against them. See *VA Health Care: Actions Needed to Improve Administration of the Provider Performance Pay and Award Systems,* GAO-13-536 (Washington, D.C.: July 24, 2013).

To examine VAMCs' reviews of providers' clinical care after concerns are raised, we reviewed VHA policies and guidance and interviewed relevant VHA officials to obtain an understanding of VHA processes for these reviews.[7] In addition, we identified providers whose clinical care required a review after concerns were raised at a non-generalizable selection of five VAMCs from October 2013 through the time we completed our site visits in March 2017. For these selected providers, we reviewed VAMC documentation of their reviews. We selected the five VAMCs based on the complexity of services offered and their geographic distribution. We identified providers at each VAMC by reviewing documentation of each VAMC's credentialing committee meetings from fiscal year 2014 through fiscal year 2016.[8] During our visits, we interviewed VAMC officials, including chiefs of staff, clinical supervisors known as service chiefs, and other officials involved in these reviews. We asked the officials to clarify information about the documentation we received and confirm the completeness of the list of providers we identified. Based on the documentation and interviews, we determined the type of reviews the selected VAMCs conducted and the extent to which the VAMCs took adverse privileging actions against any of the identified providers.[9] We assessed the extent to which the selected VAMCs adhered to VHA policy requirements for clinical care reviews and we compared these VHA policies and the selected VAMCs' reviews to federal internal control standards related to monitoring and documentation.[10] To review

---

[7] Veterans Health Administration, *Credentialing and Privileging*, VHA Handbook 1100.19 (Washington, D.C.: Oct. 15, 2012) and *Provider Competency and Clinical Care Concerns Including Focused Clinical Care Review and FPPE for Cause Guidance*, v.2 (Washington, D.C.: Jul. 2016).

[8] VAMCs generally have a committee responsible for making recommendations to VAMC leadership on matters related to credentialing and privileging, referred to in this report as the credentialing committee. Credentialing is the process of collecting and reviewing information—such as a provider's professional training, malpractice history, peer references, and other components of professional background—to determine whether the provider has suitable abilities and experience to provide medical services at a VAMC.

[9] We limited our review of adverse privileging actions to final actions—that is, when all applicable internal VAMC due process procedures have been completed.

[10] GAO, *Standards for Internal Control in the Federal Government*, GAO-14-704G (Washington, D.C.: Sept. 10, 2014) and *Standards for Internal Control in the Federal Government*, GAO/AIMD-00-21.3.1 (Washington, D.C.: Nov. 1, 1999). Internal control is a

VHA's oversight of VAMCs' clinical care reviews and adverse privileging actions, we reviewed VHA policy for oversight responsibilities and requirements. We also interviewed relevant VHA officials, as well as officials in VA's Veterans Integrated Service Networks (VISN) responsible for each of the five selected VAMCs, about their oversight activities.[11] We also compared VHA's policy and the selected VISNs' oversight activities with federal internal control standards related to monitoring.[12]

To examine VAMCs' reporting of providers to the NPDB and SLBs, we reviewed VHA's related policies and evaluated the extent to which the selected VAMCs adhered to these policies.[13] Specifically, we evaluated the extent to which providers whose clinical care required a review or resulted in the VAMC taking adverse privileging actions against them from October 2013 through the time we completed our site visits in March 2017 were reported to the NPDB and the SLBs when appropriate. Our review of NPDB reporting is limited to NPDB adverse action reports, which are reports of the adverse privileging actions VAMCs took against providers and any providers who resigned or retired while under investigation for a clinical care concern. Our review does not include VHA reporting of providers for paid medical malpractice settlements or judgements (tort claims). We reviewed VAMC documentation related to its reporting of specific providers and interviewed VAMC officials, including both clinical and administrative officials involved in these reporting processes. To examine VHA's oversight of VAMC reporting, we reviewed VHA policies for overseeing NPDB and SLB reporting and interviewed relevant VHA officials as well as officials in the VISNs responsible for each of the five selected VAMCs about VISN oversight activities. We also compared

---

process effected by an entity's management, oversight body, and other personnel that provides reasonable assurance that the objectives of an entity will be achieved.

[11] VISNs are regional systems of care that oversee the day-to-day functions of VAMCs that are within their network. Each VAMC is assigned to one of VA's 18 VISNs.

[12] GAO-14-704G and GAO/AIMD-00-21.3.1.

[13] Veterans Health Administration, *National Practitioner Data Bank (NPDB) Reports,* VHA Handbook 1100.17 (Washington, D.C.: Dec. 28, 2009); Veterans Health Administration, *Reporting and Responding to State Licensing Boards*, VHA Handbook 1100.18 (Washington, D.C.: Dec. 22, 2005); and VHA, *Credentialing and Privileging*, VHA Handbook 1100.19.

VHA's policy for oversight responsibilities and the selected VISNs' oversight activities with federal internal control standards related to monitoring.[14]

To determine the extent to which VAMCs give performance pay to providers who have had an adverse privileging action taken against them, we reviewed documentation of performance pay given to providers we identified with adverse privileging actions at the five selected VAMCs. Specifically, for each of the providers with an adverse privileging action who were eligible for performance pay, we reviewed documentation of performance pay for the fiscal year in which the action was taken and for the fiscal year prior to the action. Our performance pay analysis does not include contract providers, because only employed providers are eligible to receive performance pay.[15] We also reviewed VA policy on performance pay and interviewed relevant VHA officials, as well as VAMC officials, about performance pay.

We conducted this performance audit from August 2016 to November 2017 in accordance with generally accepted government auditing standards. Those standards require that we plan and perform the audit to obtain sufficient, appropriate evidence to provide a reasonable basis for our findings and conclusions based on our audit objectives. We believe that the evidence obtained provides a reasonable basis for our findings and conclusions based on our audit objectives.

BACKGROUND

Identifying Concerns about Providers' Clinical Care

As part of the credentialing and privileging process, VAMC officials are responsible for monitoring each provider's performance on an ongoing basis and identifying any concerns about clinical care that may warrant

---

[14] GAO-14-704G and GAO/AIMD-00-21.3.1.

[15] Department of Veterans Affairs, *Pay Administration*, VA Handbook 5007, v.52 (Washington, D.C.: Mar. 4, 2016).

further review. VAMCs can identify concerns about providers' clinical care in a variety of ways, including the following:

- Ongoing monitoring. VHA requires VAMCs to conduct and document ongoing monitoring of each provider's performance at least twice a year through an ongoing professional practice evaluation. During this evaluation, a provider's performance is evaluated against benchmarks established by VAMC leadership that define acceptable performance, such as documenting patient visits appropriately and achieving specific patient outcomes.
- Peer review triggers. VHA has a separate process, called peer review, that VAMCs may use to review adverse events.[16] While information collected as part of peer review is protected for quality improvement purposes and may not be used to take action against a provider, VAMCs can identify concerns about a provider's clinical care based on a trend of certain peer review outcomes over a specified period of time, referred to as triggers. VHA requires VAMCs to establish peer review triggers. An example of a peer review trigger is when a provider has two or more episodes of patient care within a 12- month period for which a peer determined that most experienced, competent providers would have managed the episodes differently.
- Complaints or incident reports. Concerns about a provider's clinical care can also be identified through complaints and incident reports.[17] These can come from any individual with a concern, including patients, providers, or VAMC leadership.

---

[16] Peer review is a VHA process for determining whether a provider's actions associated with an adverse event were clinically appropriate—that is, whether another provider with similar expertise would have taken similar action. Adverse events are clinical incidents that may pose a risk of injury to a patient and result from a medical intervention or lack of an appropriate intervention, such as a missed or delayed diagnosis, rather than from the patient's underlying medical condition.

[17] Each VAMC maintains its own incident reporting system, which is used by VAMC staff to report adverse events. Adverse events also include nonclinical incidents, such as reported thefts or conflicts between employees; such incidences would not likely result in a concern being raised about a provider's clinical care. In addition to reviewing providers' clinical care, VAMCs have other processes available to them for responding to an adverse event or

- Tort claims. Filed or settled tort claims or malpractice claims can raise a concern about a provider not identified through ongoing monitoring or peer review.

Reviewing Concerns about Providers' Clinical Care and Taking Adverse Privileging Actions

Once a concern about a provider's clinical care is identified, VHA policy and guidance establish processes for VAMC officials to use to review the concern and determine whether an action should be taken against the provider's clinical privileges. VHA policy states that if allowing a provider under review to continue delivering patient care could result in imminent danger to veterans, VAMC officials should remove the provider from delivering patient care through a summary suspension of privileges. VAMC officials have flexibility to determine the most appropriate process to use to review a provider's clinical care depending on the specific concerns and the situation. These processes include the following:

- Focused professional practice evaluation (FPPE) for cause. This is a prospective review of the provider's care over a specified period of time, during which the provider has the opportunity to demonstrate improvement in the specific area of concern. Failure to improve could result in further review or action.
- Retrospective review. This is a review of the provider's delivery of patient care focused on a specific period of time in the past, a specific area of practice, or both, based on an identified concern.
- Comprehensive review. This is a more extensive retrospective review, generally performed by a panel of experts to ensure fairness and objectivity. In addition to reviewing the provider's

---

incident report. For more information about these other processes, see GAO, *Veterans Health Care: Veterans Health Administration Processes for Responding to Reported Adverse Events*, GAO-12-827R (Washington, D.C.: Aug. 24, 2012).

past patient care, these reviews may also include interviews with the provider, patients, and staff. These reviews generally result in conclusions about whether care delivered by the provider met the standard of care and may include recommendations about the provider's privileges.

Once a review is completed, VAMC leadership officials and the VAMC credentialing committee make decisions about next steps, which could include the following:

- do nothing, if the review did not substantiate the concerns;
- conduct further review (such as an FPPE for cause to allow the provider an opportunity for improvement or a comprehensive review if more information is needed); or
- take an adverse privileging action, including limiting one or more privileges (such as prescribing medication or performing a certain procedure) or revoking all of the provider's privileges.

If the VAMC's credentialing committee recommends an adverse privileging action, it is the VAMC director's responsibility to weigh all available information, including recommendations, and take an action. After a permanent provider is notified of the director's decision, the provider can appeal the decision to the Disciplinary Appeals Board as part of their due process rights.[18] The adverse privileging action is considered final once the Disciplinary Appeals Board reaches a decision and the Deputy Under Secretary for Health executes the Board's decision.[19] If a permanent provider does not make use of the offered due process procedures within 7 days, the provider waives his or her right to due process and the adverse privileging action is considered final.

---

[18] Due process varies by appointment type, with non-permanent providers having access to a limited fair hearing to determine if the reason for the adverse privileging action was related to substandard care, professional misconduct, or professional incompetence. Non-permanent providers cannot internally appeal the adverse privileging action itself.

[19] A provider adversely affected by a decision of the Disciplinary Appeals Board (as reviewed by the Secretary) may obtain judicial review of the decision. 38 U.S.C. § 7462(f)(1).

Reporting Providers to the NPDB and SLBs

VHA policy requires VAMCs to alert certain entities if there are serious concerns with regard to a provider's clinical performance. VHA policy assigns reporting responsibility and authority to the VAMC director, who generally delegates the task of reporting to other VAMC officials. VHA makes this information available to other health care entities through two distinct reporting processes:

NPDB

Under VHA policy, VAMC directors must report to the NPDB any adverse privileging action the facility takes that 1) affects the clinical privileges of a provider for a period longer than 30 days and 2) is related to professional incompetence or professional misconduct.[20] VHA policy requires VAMCs to submit these NPDB adverse action reports within 15 calendar days of the date the adverse privileging action is made final— that is, when all applicable internal due process procedures have been completed and the VAMC director has signed off on the action. VAMC directors are also required to report to the NPDB providers who resign or retire while under investigation or in return for the VAMC not conducting such an investigation or proceeding.[21] To avoid any errors in the facts of

---

[20] VHA policy also requires VAMCs to forward a copy of the NPDB report to the SLB(s) where the provider holds an active medical license and to the SLB where the VAMC is located if the provider does not hold a license in that state. VA policy requires that providers hold one active unrestricted state medical license and does not require the provider to be licensed in the state where the VAMC is located. The Health Care Quality Improvement Act of 1986, which called for the establishment of the NPDB and requires the reporting of certain information, including information on professional review actions taken by health care entities, also required VA and the Department of Health and Human Services to enter into a memorandum of understanding regarding VA's reporting of such information. In 1990 the two agencies entered into such an understanding, and VHA policy lays out these agreed upon reporting procedures for VAMCs. See Pub. L. No. 99-600, Tit. IV, 100 Stat. 3743, 3784 (1986), codified, as amended, at 42 U.S.C. §§ 11101-11152). VA's updated reporting procedures are found at 38 C.F.R. Part 46.

[21] The NPDB defines an investigation broadly, running from the start of an inquiry until a final decision on an adverse privileging action is reached. An investigation must be focused on the provider in question, must concern the professional conduct or professional competence of the provider in question, and generally should be a precursor to a final action. According to VHA guidance, FPPEs for cause are not considered an investigation or a clinical

the report, the VAMC director must notify any provider who is about to be reported to the NPDB and give the provider an opportunity to discuss the content of the report before it is submitted.

SLBs

VHA policy requires VAMC directors to report providers—both current and former employees—when there are serious concerns about the providers' clinical care to any SLB where the providers hold an active medical license.

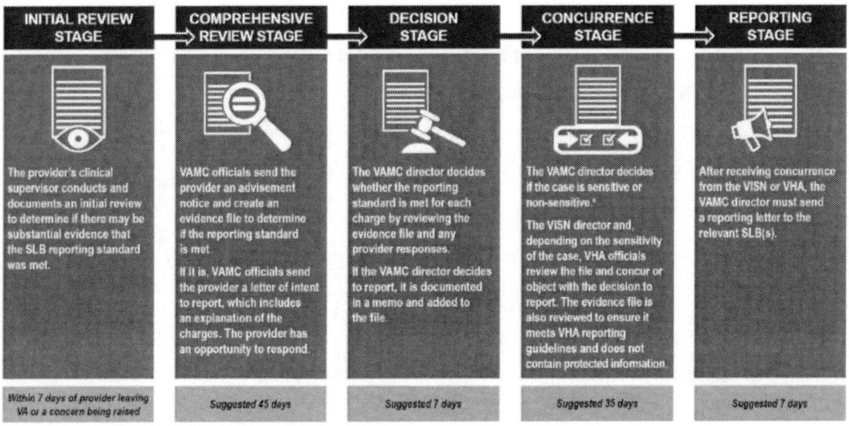

Legend: SLB = state licensing board; VAMC = Department of Veterans Affairs medical center; VISN = Veterans Integrated Service Network.

Source: GAO review of VHA policy. | GAO-18-63

[a] A case is considered sensitive if (a) it includes a previous history of licensure action against the provider; (b) it includes the death of a patient; (c) the provider has retained legal counsel in anticipation of litigation; (d) there has been media attention related to some aspect of the case; or (e) the provider has a clinical diagnosis, or is under the care of a physician, and that information is part of the review or provider response includes the provider's personal health information.

Figure 1. An Overview of the Stages of the Veterans Health Administration's (VHA) State Licensing Board Reporting Process.

---

privileging action and thus a provider would not be reported for resigning or retiring during an FPPE for cause.

Specifically, VHA policy requires VAMCs to report providers who so substantially failed to meet generally accepted standards of clinical practice as to raise reasonable concern for the safety of patients. According to VHA policy and guidance, the SLB reporting process should be initiated as soon as it appears that a provider's behavior or clinical practice fails to meet accepted standards. VAMC officials are directed not to wait to report to SLBs until adverse privileging actions are taken because an SLB conducts its own investigation of the provider to determine whether licensure action is warranted. This chaptering process comprises five stages as established in VHA policy, and VHA policy states that the process should be completed in around 100 days (see Figure 1).

Performance Pay

Performance pay—a component of VA provider compensation—is an annual lump sum payment based on the extent to which an individual provider achieves specific goals. The goals may vary for providers across VA, at the same VAMC, or within a particular specialty. VA policy establishes minimum performance pay eligibility criteria, including being employed by VA from July 1 through September 30 of the fiscal year being reviewed.

Selected VAMCs' Reviews of Providers' Clinical Care Are Not Always Documented or Timely, and VHA Does Not Adequately Oversee these Reviews

Documentation Frequently Lacking

We found that the five selected VAMCs collectively required reviews of 148 providers' clinical care after concerns were raised from October 2013 through March 2017, but VAMC officials were unable to provide documentation that almost half of these reviews were conducted. We found that all five VAMCs lacked at least some documentation of the reviews they told us they conducted, and in some cases the required reviews were not conducted at all. We also found VHA does not adequately oversee these reviews, as discussed later in this chapter.

- FPPEs for cause. FPPEs for cause accounted for most of the missing documentation of clinical care reviews, despite VHA policy requiring VAMCs to document FPPEs for cause in the providers' files. Specifically, of the 112 providers for whom the selected VAMCs required FPPEs for cause from October 2013 through March 2017, the VAMCs were unable to provide documentation of the FPPEs for nearly a quarter (26) of the providers. Additionally, VAMC officials confirmed that FPPEs for cause that were required for another 21 providers were never conducted.
- Other reviews. The selected VAMCs were also unable to provide documentation of some retrospective reviews. Specifically, of the 27 providers for whom the selected VAMCs conducted a retrospective review, 8 were missing documentation. While VHA guidance recommends that VAMCs document these reviews, VHA policy does not require that VAMCs document retrospective or comprehensive reviews. VHA officials told us that they expected VAMCs to document these types of reviews so that the information could be used to support adverse privileging actions, if necessary. Without clearly stated documentation requirements in VHA policy, VAMC officials inconsistently document their results, preventing VAMC directors and VISNs from properly evaluating the effectiveness of its retrospective and comprehensive reviews, which are used to, among other things, ensure patient safety. Additionally, we found that key officials from two VAMCs were not aware of the VHA guidance and that 5 of the 8 missing retrospective reviews were from these two VAMCs.

  We also found that one VAMC was missing documentation of clinical care reviews for 12 providers who met the VAMC's peer review trigger. In the absence of this documentation, we were unable to identify the type of reviews that were missing for these 12 providers.

The selected VAMCs' failure to document reviews of providers' clinical care after concerns were raised is inconsistent with federal internal control standards for monitoring and documentation, which state that management should conduct and document separate evaluations, when necessary.[22] In the absence of VAMC documentation of such separate evaluations of providers, VAMC leadership officials lack key information needed to make decisions about whether providers' privileges are appropriate, and they also lack reasonable assurance that appropriate reviews are conducted.

Reviews Not Always Timely

We found that the five selected VAMCs' reviews of providers' clinical care were not always conducted in a timely manner after concerns were raised. Specifically, of the 148 providers, the VAMCs' initiation of reviews of 16 providers' clinical care was delayed by more than 3 months, and in some cases for multiple years, after the concern was raised.[23] At one VAMC, service chiefs were not instructed to conduct reviews of 14 providers until 4 to 13 months after these providers met the VAMC's peer review trigger.[24] Before the service chiefs were notified of the concerns, 3 of these providers had at least one additional concerning episode of care—that peer reviewers judged would have been handled differently by most experienced providers—identified through the peer review process.[25] As

[22] GAO-14-704G and GAO/AIMD-00-21.3.1.

[23] VHA policy and guidance do not specify how quickly a clinical care review should be initiated after a concern is identified. We define a delay as longer than 3 months because FPPEs for cause are generally completed within this timeframe.

[24] For 1 of the 14 providers, the service chief became aware that the provider met a peer review trigger and conducted a review before the notification letter was sent.

[25] One provider had two additional concerning episodes of care before the service chief was notified that the provider met the peer review trigger.

pointed out in VHA guidance, earlier intervention could prevent additional patients from receiving substandard care. Officials from another VAMC did not conduct retrospective reviews on 2 providers until we requested documentation of the reviews, approximately 3 and a half years after the credentialing committee had initially requested a review.[26]

While VHA officials told us that clinical care reviews should be conducted as expeditiously as reasonably possible, VHA policy does not specify a timeliness requirement. Allowing more time to elapse before a clinical care review is initiated weakens the intended purpose behind clinical care reviews and further increases risk to patient safety. Federal internal control standards for monitoring state that management should evaluate issues and remediate identified deficiencies in a timely manner.[27]A clinical care concern could represent a potential deficiency in providing medical care, and as a result, VHA increases its risk further without establishing a policy that sets timeframes for conducting clinical care reviews.

VHA Oversight is Inadequate

We also found that VHA does not adequately oversee VAMC reviews of providers' clinical care after concerns have been raised, including ensuring that these reviews are completed and documented in a timely manner. Under VHA policy, VISNs are responsible for overseeing the credentialing and privileging processes at their respective VAMCs. While reviews of providers' clinical care after concerns are raised are a component of credentialing and privileging, we found that the VISNs with responsibility for overseeing the selected VAMCs through routine audits do not include these reviews in their audits. While the standardized tool VHA requires the VISNs to use for these audits instructs the VISNs to identify and review providers who were on an FPPE for cause, none of the VISN officials we spoke with described any routine oversight of FPPEs or

[26] The reviews did not identify any additional clinical care concerns.
[27] GAO-14-704G and GAO/AIMD-00-21.3.1.

any other reviews of identified clinical care concerns.[28] This may be in part because some VISN officials are not using VHA's standardized audit tool as required. Officials from one VISN said they had developed their own audit tool and officials from another VISN said that they were not conducting the audits due to multiple instances of turnover in a key position at the VISN. Further, VHA's standardized audit tool does not direct the VISN to oversee any other types of reviews of clinical care concerns, such as retrospective or comprehensive reviews. The tool also does not require VISN officials to look at documentation of the FPPEs for cause; instead, it calls for reviewing credentialing committee meeting minutes. Without reviewing documentation, VISN officials would be unable to identify the incomplete documentation that we identified in our review. Both VHA and VISN officials described instances of assisting VAMC officials with reviews of providers' clinical care after concerns had been raised, but VHA and VISN officials told us that their involvement in these reviews is typically consultative and not routine. (For example, the VISN may assist by identifying providers outside of the VAMC to conduct the review.) As a result, VHA and the VISNs are not conducting routine oversight to ensure that VAMC reviews of providers' clinical care after concerns are raised are conducted appropriately, including adequately ensuring that the reviews are completed and documented in a timely manner, in accordance with VHA policy.

The lack of routine VHA oversight, through the VISNs, of VAMC reviews of providers' clinical care after concerns are raised is inconsistent with federal internal control standards for monitoring, which state that management should establish and operate monitoring activities.[29] In the absence of routine monitoring of VAMCs' evaluations of providers after concerns have been raised, VHA lacks reasonable assurance that VAMCs adequately review all identified concerns about providers' clinical care and

---

[28] Regarding their audits of VAMCs, VISN officials we interviewed generally described selecting a sample of providers from different specialties to review VAMC compliance with other, more routine credentialing and privileging requirements, such as appropriate verification of licensure. Some officials said they would look at documentation of a VAMC's review of a provider's clinical care after a concern had been raised if any of the providers in their sample happened to have a documented review in their files.

[29] GAO-14-704G and GAO/AIMD-00-21.3.1.

take appropriate privileging actions to ensure that VA is providing safe, high quality care for veterans.

SELECTED VAMCS DID NOT ALWAYS REPORT PROVIDERS TO THE NPDB AND SLBS IN ACCORDANCE WITH VHA POLICY, AND VHA DOES NOT ADEQUATELY OVERSEE THIS REPORTING

NPDB and SLB Reporting Not Completed

We found that the five selected VAMCs did not report the majority of providers who should have been reported to the NPDB or SLBs in accordance with VHA policy.[30] Our analysis shows that from October 2013 through March 2017, of the 148 providers whose clinical care required a review, the VAMCs took adverse privileging actions against 5 providers, and another 4 providers resigned or retired while under review but before an adverse privileging action could be taken. However, at the time of our review, we found that the five selected VAMCs had only reported 1 of these 9 providers to the NPDB and none of these providers to the SLBs.[31] Furthermore, the 1 provider who was reported to the NPDB for an adverse privileging action was reported 136 days after all internal VA appeals were complete, far beyond the 15 day reporting requirement.

In addition to these nine providers, one of the selected VAMCs terminated the services of four contract providers based on deficiencies in the providers' clinical performance, effectively revoking their clinical privileges. For example, the VAMC documented that one contractor's

[30] Statements about SLB reporting in this report refer to the requirement that VAMC directors report to SLBs those providers who so substantially failed to meet generally accepted standards of clinical practice as to raise reasonable concern for the safety of patients, unless otherwise stated. This requirement is separate from the requirement that a copy of an NPDB report of an adverse privileging action be provided to any SLB where the provider holds an active medical license and to the SLB where the VAMC is located if the provider does not hold a license in that state. It is assumed that if a provider was not reported to the NPDB, a copy of such a report could not have been provided to the appropriate SLBs.

[31] Officials documented that these nine providers met the standard for reporting to the SLB after they separated from the VAMC.

services were terminated for cause related to patient abuse after only 2 weeks of work at the VAMC. A VAMC leadership official told us there was no further documentation of whether reporting was considered or whether any comprehensive review was conducted, despite the fact that the VAMC credentialing committee recommended both. While VHA policy identifies the requirements, steps, and limited fair hearing process for reporting contract providers, these required steps were not followed, and none of these providers were reported to the NPDB or SLB.

As a result of our audit work, in August 2017, one of the VAMCs reported to the NPDB three of the providers who resigned or retired while under investigation but before an adverse privileging action could be taken. These reports were completed between 11 months and over 3 and a half years after the providers resigned or retired. VAMC officials could not confirm that they sent the required copies of the NPDB reports to the appropriate SLBs.

The five selected VAMCs did report two providers to their respective SLBs for reasons other than adverse privileging actions. In accordance with VHA policy, these SLB reports were made after VAMC officials determined that the providers' behavior or clinical practice so substantially failed to meet generally accepted standards of clinical practice as to raise reasonable concern for the safety of patients—the standard for SLB reporting. One of these providers could not have an adverse privileging action taken against them because VAMC officials unintentionally allowed the provider's privileges to expire during a comprehensive review of the provider's care. The other provider reported to the SLBs was considered for an adverse privileging action, but VAMC officials suspended the provider instead. The provider demonstrated improvement after the suspension.

SLB Reporting Not Always Timely

While two of the selected VAMCs had each reported a provider, we found that in these cases the SLB reporting process took significantly longer than the 100 day timeframe suggested in VHA policy. Specifically, it took over 500 days for each of the two completed reports to pass initial and comprehensive review at the VAMC, receive concurrence from the VISN, and be submitted to the SLB. For example, one of the two providers self-reported to the SLB the concerning episode of care at the VAMC. However, before the VAMC submitted its SLB report 328 days later, the SLB had completed its investigation of the provider's self-report and put in place an agreement that placed restrictions and requirements on the provider's medical license. Subsequently, the provider successfully met the requirements of the agreement and had all restrictions on the license removed. Officials at two VAMCs told us the SLB reporting is more tedious or cumbersome than the NPDB reporting process, making it difficult to complete in a timely manner. One VAMC official commented that while completing the process in less than a year seems reasonable, the typical timeframe for submitting a SLB report is at least 2 years.

At the five selected VAMCs, we found that providers were not reported to the NPDB and relevant SLBs as required because officials were generally not familiar with or misinterpreted related VHA policies. VHA officials commented that adverse privileging actions and clinical care concerns rising to the level of reporting are infrequent, with officials at two VISNs estimating that only a few occur across the facilities within their network each year. Staff at three VAMCs commented that there has been turnover in positions that have been delegated tasks related to reporting and one VAMC official told us that turnover in these positions is a barrier to timely reporting. For example,

- at one facility, we found that officials failed to report six providers to the NPDB because the officials were unaware that they had been delegated responsibility for NPDB reporting.[32]
- Officials at two of the selected VAMCs told us that VHA cannot report contract providers to the NPDB. This assertion is inconsistent with VHA policy.

---

[32] After our review, VAMC officials reported three of these six providers to the NPDB.

- Officials at two of the selected VAMCs were waiting to start the SLB reporting process for providers until after all appeals had been exhausted. This approach is inconsistent with VHA policy, which states that the process should start within 7 days of when the reporting standard is met. For example, for one provider who was reported, VAMC officials unnecessarily waited 7 months for the completion of the appeals process before they resumed the reporting process, which ultimately took 547 days.
- Officials at one VAMC did not report a provider to the NPDB or SLB following an adverse privileging action because the SLB had found out about the issue independently. This is inconsistent with VHA policy for NPDB and SLB reporting, and the SLBs in other states where the provider held a license were not alerted of concerns about the provider's clinical practice.

VHA Oversight is Inadequate

We also found that VHA and the VISNs do not adequately oversee NPDB and SLB reporting and they cannot ensure that VAMCs are reporting providers when required to do so by VHA policy. While the VISNs are responsible for overseeing the credentialing and privileging at their respective VAMCs under VHA policy, VHA policy does not require the VISNs to oversee whether VAMCs are reporting providers to the NPDB or SLB when warranted. As a result, VISN officials were unaware of situations in which VAMC directors failed to report providers to the NPDB, as evidenced by our review. In the case of reporting processes for SLBs, VISN officials told us that they review the evidence files to ensure, among other things, that the files are in compliance with privacy laws. However, officials told us that the VISNs do not oversee the reporting process to ensure that VAMC directors are reporting all providers to the SLB who should be reported. Additionally, VHA officials told us that they are not aware of the number of cases that have been initiated for SLB reporting.

Further, by failing to report providers as required, VHA facilitates providers who provide substandard care obtaining privileges at another VAMC or a hospital outside of VA's health care system without an indication on their record that an adverse privileging action was taken against them or that they resigned or retired while under investigation. For example, we found that

- two of the four contract providers whose privileges were revoked and were not reported to the NPDB or SLBs by one VAMC continue to be able to provide care to veterans outside of that VAMC. Specifically, one provider whose services were terminated related to patient abuse subsequently held privileges at another VAMC, while the other provider belongs to a network of providers that provides care for veterans in the community.[33]
- Seven of the 12 providers who were not reported to the NPDB or SLBs after their privileges were revoked—through adverse privileging actions or the termination of services on a contract—or who resigned or retired while under investigation have current Medicare enrollment records, indicating that they are likely practicing outside of VA and may still be receiving federal dollars by billing for services provided to Medicare beneficiaries.
- We also identified one case where a VAMC director did not report a provider to the NPDB or SLB after an agreement was reached that the provider would resign, though the VAMC credentialing committee recommended the provider's privileges be revoked. We found that the provider's privileges were also revoked from a non-VA hospital in the same city for the same reason 2 years later. The director's decision not to report the provider as required left patients in that community vulnerable to adverse outcomes

[33] The Patient-Centered Community Care and Veterans Choice programs are two of VA's programs that allow eligible veterans to receive care in the community when generally (1) its medical facilities do not offer the services needed on site, (2) the veteran would have to travel a long distance to obtain care from a VHA medical facility, or (3) there are long wait times to obtain appointments at VHA medical facilities. Under both programs, VA's two third party administrators are responsible for developing regional networks of providers to deliver care to eligible veterans.

because problems with the provider's performance were not disclosed. There was no documentation of the reasons why the VAMC director did not report the provider to the NPDB or SLBs.[34]

This lack of routine oversight from VHA through the VISNs of VAMCs' reporting of providers to the NPDB and SLBs is inconsistent with federal internal control standards for monitoring. The standards state that management should establish and operate monitoring activities to monitor the internal control system and appropriately remediate deficiencies on a timely basis.[35] Without routine monitoring of the reporting process, VHA lacks reasonable assurance that all providers who should be reported to the NPDB and SLBs are reported.

AT SELECTED VAMCS, PROVIDERS WITH ADVERSE PRIVILEGING ACTIONS WERE INELIGIBLE FOR PERFORMANCE PAY THE YEAR THE ACTIONS WERE TAKEN

None of the five providers who had an adverse privileging action taken against them in the period we reviewed received performance pay for the fiscal year the action was taken because they were ineligible, per VA policy.[36] This is because VA policy requires providers to be employed through the end of the fiscal year to be eligible for performance pay, and none of the five providers we reviewed were still employed by the VAMCs at the end of the fiscal year in which the actions were taken.

All five of the adverse privileging actions resulted from concerns about the providers' clinical care in previous fiscal years. Among the five providers, two providers received performance pay in the fiscal year before

[34] We were unable to interview the VAMC director because he had retired.

[35] GAO-14-704G and GAO/AIMD-00-21.3.1.

[36] Since contract providers are not eligible for performance pay, our review of performance pay did not include the four providers that one VAMC released from their contracts based on substandard care.

their privileges were revoked, and three providers did not. For example, one provider's privileges were revoked in 2015 due to concerns raised in 2014 regarding the provider's failure to complete necessary documentation of patient care in a timely manner. This provider did not receive credit for the performance pay goal directly related to timely completion of documentation, and ultimately the provider received half of the maximum amount of performance pay for fiscal year 2014. In the case of another provider who did not receive any performance pay for the fiscal year before the adverse privileging action was taken, VAMC officials noted that the provider had been removed from practice for a portion of the fiscal year while they were reviewing the clinical care concern and thus was unable to meet performance pay goals.

CONCLUSIONS

VHA is responsible for ensuring that providers at its VAMCs deliver safe care to veterans and that concerns that may arise about providers' clinical care are reviewed and addressed at VHA's 170 VAMCs. However, our work shows that at our five selected VAMCs, reviews of concerns about providers' clinical care were not always documented or conducted in a timely manner and VAMCs had not reported the majority of providers they should have reported to the NPDB or SLBs. This is concerning for several reasons. First, without documentation of the reviews of these concerns about providers' clinical care, VAMC leadership officials may not have the information they need to make decisions about whether a provider's privileges at the VAMC are appropriate. Second, if VAMCs do not document that they have reviewed provider's clinical care after concerns have been raised, VHA lacks reasonable assurance that the VAMCs are adequately addressing such concerns or that VAMCs are limiting or revoking providers' privileges when necessary. Third, if these reviews are not conducted in a timely manner and providers continue to deliver potentially substandard care, VHA may be increasing the risk that veterans will receive unsafe care at VAMCs. Finally, VAMCs' failure to report providers to the NPDB and SLBs, as required under VHA policy, makes it possible for providers to obtain privileges at other VAMCs or non-VA health care entities without disclosing the problems with their past performance. In effect, this can help shield the providers from professional accountability outside of VA's health care system.

Further, VHA's inadequate oversight of these processes calls into question the extent to which VAMCs are held accountable for ensuring that veterans receive safe, high quality care. As our review shows, the VISNs responsible for overseeing the five selected VAMCs do not routinely oversee VAMC reviews of providers' clinical care after concerns are raised to ensure that these reviews are completed in accordance with VHA policies; nor do the VISNs oversee the VAMCs to ensure that all providers that should be reported are reported to the NPDB and SLBs. Until VHA strengthens its oversight of these processes, veterans may be at increased risk of receiving unsafe care through the VA health care system.

RECOMMENDATIONS FOR EXECUTIVE ACTION

We are making the following four recommendations to VA:

The Under Secretary for Health should specify in VHA policy that reviews of providers' clinical care after concerns have been raised should be documented, including retrospective and comprehensive reviews. (Recommendation 1)

The Under Secretary for Health should specify in VHA policy a timeliness requirement for initiating reviews of providers' clinical care after a concern has been raised. (Recommendation 2)

The Under Secretary for Health should require VISN officials to oversee VAMC reviews of providers' clinical care after concerns have been raised, including retrospective and comprehensive reviews, and ensure that VISN officials are conducting such oversight with the required standardized audit tool. This oversight should include reviewing documentation in order to ensure that these reviews are documented appropriately and conducted in a timely manner. (Recommendation 3)

The Under Secretary for Health should require VISN officials to establish a process for overseeing VAMCs to ensure that they are reporting providers to the NPDB and SLBs, and are reporting in a timely manner. (Recommendation 4)

AGENCY COMMENTS

We provided a draft of this chapter to VA for comment. In its written comments, which are reproduced in Appendix I, VA agreed with our conclusions and concurred with our recommendations. In its comments, VA stated that VHA plans to revise existing policy to require documentation of reviews of providers' clinical care after concerns have been raised and to establish expected timeframes for completing such reviews. VA estimates that it will complete these actions by September 2018. VA also stated that VHA will update the standardized audit tool used by the VISNs so that it directs them to oversee reviews of providers' clinical care after concerns have been raised and to ensure timely reporting to the NPDB and SLBs. According to VA, the revised tool will also facilitate aggregate reporting by VISNs to identify trends and issues. VA estimates that it will complete these actions by October 2018.

As agreed with your office, unless you publicly announce the contents of this chapter earlier, we plan no further distribution until 30 days from the report date. At that time, we will send copies to the appropriate congressional committees, the Secretary of Veterans Affairs, and the Under Secretary for Health.

Sincerely yours,

Sharon M. Silas
Acting Director, Health Care

Randall B. Williamson
Director, Health Care

Appendix I: Comments from the Department of Veterans Affairs

DEPARTMENT OF VETERANS AFFAIRS
WASHINGTON DC 20420

October 20, 2017

Mr. Randall B. Williamson
Director, Health Care
U.S. Government Accountability Office
441 G Street, NW
Washington, DC 20548

Dear Mr. Williamson:

The Department of Veterans Affairs (VA) has reviewed the Government Accountability Office's (GAO) draft report, ***"VA HEALTH CARE: Improved Policies and Oversight Needed for Reviewing and Reporting Providers for Quality and Safety Concerns"*** (GAO-18-63). VA agrees with GAO's conclusions and concurs with GAO's recommendations to the Department.

The enclosure provides information on actions taken to address the GAO draft report recommendations.

VA appreciates the opportunity to comment on your draft report.

Sincerely,

Gina S. Farrisee
Deputy Chief of Staff

Department of Veterans Affairs (VA) Comments to
Government Accountability Office (GAO) Draft Report
"VA HEALTH CARE: Improved Policies and Oversight Needed for Reviewing and Reporting Providers for Quality and Safety Concerns"
(GAO-18-63)

Recommendation 1: The Under Secretary for Health should specify in VHA policy that reviews of providers' clinical care after concerns are raised should be documented, including retrospective and comprehensive reviews.

VA Comment: Concur. The Veterans Health Administration's (VHA) Office of Quality, Safety, and Value, Medical Staff Affairs, will rewrite policy to formalize guidance on focused management reviews that are to be conducted when a clinical care concern has been raised. Policy will codify maintenance of these reviews in the Provider Profile and in accordance with the System of Records Notice 77VA10A4, "Health Care Provider Credentialing and Privileging Records – VA." Existing policy will be expanded to incorporate existing guidance documents related to the process of addressing clinical care concerns for privileged providers to facilitate standardization throughout the agency. The Assistant Deputy Under Secretary for Clinical Operations will review and facilitate the distribution of interim guidance by December 2017 related to addressing clinical care concerns for privileged providers which will include documentation and maintenance of focused management reviews. This process has a target completion date of September 2018.

Recommendation 2: The Under Secretary for Health should specify in VHA policy a timeliness requirement for initiating reviews of providers' clinical care after a concern is raised.

VA Comment: Concur. VHA's Office of Quality, Safety, and Value, Medical Staff Affairs will rewrite policy to include timeline expectations for initiating a focused management review when a clinical care concern has been triggered for a privileged provider. Existing policy will be expanded to incorporate existing guidance documents related to the process of addressing clinical care concerns for privileged providers to facilitate standardization throughout the agency. The Assistant Deputy Under Secretary for Clinical Operations will review and facilitate the distribution of interim guidance by December 2017 related to addressing clinical care concerns for privileged providers which will include documentation and maintenance of focused management reviews. This process has a target completion date of September 2018.

Recommendation 3: The Under Secretary for Health should require VISN officials to oversee VAMC reviews of providers' clinical care after concerns are raised, including retrospective and comprehensive reviews, and ensure that VISN officials are conducting such oversight with the required standardized audit tool. This oversight should include reviewing documentation in order to ensure that these reviews are documented appropriately and conducted in a timely manner.

VA Comment: Concur. VHA's Office of Quality, Safety, and Value, Medical Staff Affairs will update the standardized auditing tool that is to be utilized by the Veterans Integrated Service Network (VISN) Chief Medical Officers to include monitoring of appropriate action taken when a facility identifies a clinical care concern with a privileged provider. The VISN auditing tool will be revised by the end of the first quarter of fiscal year (FY) 2018 and will have a reporting structure to facilitate aggregate reporting to identify trends and issues. Oversight will be demonstrated through the resulting aggregate report at the end of FY 2018, which will be produced by VHA's Office of Quality, Safety, and Value, Medical Staff Affairs. This process has a target completion date of October 2018.

Recommendation 4: The Under Secretary for Health should require VISN officials to establish a process overseeing VAMCs to ensure that they are reporting providers to the NPDB and SLBs, and are reporting in a timely manner.

VA Comment: Concur. VHA's Office of Quality, Safety, and Value, Medical Staff Affairs will update the standardized auditing tool that is to be utilized by the VISN Chief Medical Officers to include monitoring of timely reporting to National Practitioner Data Bank in accordance with VHA Handbook 1100.17, National Practitioner Data Bank, specifically for adverse privileging actions and resignation while under investigation. The tool will also incorporate monitoring of timely reporting to state licensing boards when a facility has substantial evidence that a licensed provider has failed to meet the generally accepted standard of care. The VISN auditing tool will be revised by the end of the first quarter of FY 2018 and will have a reporting structure to facilitate aggregate reporting to identify trends and issues. Oversight will be demonstrated through the resulting aggregate report at the end of FY 2018, which will be produced by VHA's Office of Quality, Safety, and Value, Medical Staff Affairs. This process has a target completion date of October 2018.

In: Improvements Needed in the VA ... ISBN: 978-1-53615-971-4
Editor: Charles Copeland

Chapter 2

IMPROVED OVERSIGHT NEEDED FOR REVIEWING AND REPORTING PROVIDERS FOR QUALITY AND SAFETY CONCERNS*

United States Government Accountability Office

Chairman Bergman, Ranking Member Kuster, and Members of the Subcommittee:

I am pleased to be here today to discuss our recent report on provider quality and safety concerns at the Department of Veterans Affairs (VA).[1] VA's Veterans Health Administration (VHA) operates one of the largest health care systems in the nation, and nearly 40,000 providers hold privileges at its 170 VA medical centers.[2] Like other health care facilities, VA medical centers are responsible for ensuring that their providers deliver

---

* This is an edited, reformatted and augmented version of United States Government Accountability Office; Report to Congressional Requesters, Publication No. GAO-18-260T, dated November 2017.

[1] GAO, *VA Health Care: Improved Policies and Oversight Needed for Reviewing and Reporting Providers for Quality and Safety* Concerns, GAO-18-63 (Washington, D.C.: Nov. 15, 2017).

[2] Privileges are the specific set of clinical services that a provider is approved to perform independently at a medical facility, based on an assessment of the provider's professional performance, judgement, clinical competence, and skills. For the purposes of this testimony, we use the term "provider" to refer to physicians and dentists.

safe care to patients. As part of this responsibility, VA medical centers are required to investigate and, if warranted, address any concerns that may arise about the clinical care their providers deliver. Concerns about a provider's clinical care can be raised for many reasons, ranging from providers not adequately documenting information about a patient's visit to practicing in a manner that is unsafe or inconsistent with industry standards of care. If VA medical centers fail to properly review and address concerns that have been raised about their providers, they may be exposing veterans to unsafe care.

Depending on the nature of the concern and the findings from their review, VA medical center officials may take adverse privileging actions against providers that either limit the care the providers are allowed to deliver at the facility or prevent the providers from delivering care altogether. VA medical center officials are required to report the providers against whom they take adverse privileging actions to the National Practitioner Data Bank (NPDB). The NPDB is used by other VA medical centers, non-VA hospitals, and other health care entities to obtain information on a provider's history of substandard care and misconduct.[3] VA medical center officials are also required to report providers to state licensing boards when there are serious concerns about the providers' clinical care. State licensing boards can then investigate and determine if the providers' conduct or ability to deliver care warrants action against the providers' medical license.

My testimony today summarizes the findings from the report, which analyzed the implementation and oversight of VHA processes for reviewing and reporting providers after quality and safety concerns have

[3] The NPDB is an electronic repository administered by the U.S. Department of Health and Human Services that collects and releases information on providers who either have been disciplined by a state licensing board, professional society, or health care entity, such as a hospital, or have been named in a medical malpractice settlement or judgment. Industry standards call for health care entities to query the NPDB and verify with the appropriate state licensing board that a provider's medical licenses are current and in good standing before appointing a provider to its medical staff and when renewing the provider's clinical privileges.

been raised at selected VA medical centers. Accordingly, this testimony addresses:

1. VA medical centers' reviews of providers' clinical care after concerns are raised and VHA's oversight of these reviews, and
2. VA medical centers' reporting of providers to the NPDB and state licensing boards and VHA's oversight of these processes.

To conduct our work, we reviewed VHA policies and guidance related to reviewing and reporting clinical care concerns about providers and interviewed relevant VHA officials. We also visited a nongeneralizable selection of five VA medical centers, selected based on the complexity of the medical services they offer veterans and to achieve variation in geography. At each VA medical center we reviewed documentation and interviewed medical center staff to 1) identify providers whose clinical care was reviewed after a concern was raised about that care and 2) determine whether the VA medical center took an adverse privileging action against any of these identified providers. In addition, we evaluated the extent to which each medical center adhered to applicable VHA policies from October 2013 through the time we completed our site visits in March 2017. We also interviewed officials from the five Veterans Integrated Service Networks (networks) that oversee the five selected medical centers. We compared VHA and the networks' oversight of the VA medical centers' reviewing and reporting of providers to VHA's related policy requirements and to federal standards for internal control related to monitoring.[4] Further details on our scope and methodology are included in our report.[5] The work this statement is based on was performed in accordance with generally accepted government auditing standards.

---

[4] GAO, *Standards for Internal Control in the Federal Government*, GAO-14-704G (Washington, D.C.: Sept. 10, 2014) and *Standards for Internal Control in the Federal Government*, GAO/AIMD-00-21.3.1 (Washington, D.C.: Nov. 1, 1999). Internal control is a process effected by an entity's management, oversight body, and other personnel that provides reasonable assurance that the objectives of an entity will be achieved.

[5] See GAO-18-63.

Selected VA Medical Centers' Reviews of Providers' Clinical Care Were Not Always Documented or Timely

We found that from October 2013 through March 2017, the five selected VA medical centers required reviews of a total of 148 providers' clinical care after concerns were raised about their care, but officials at these medical centers could not provide documentation to show that almost half of these reviews were conducted. We found that all five VA medical centers lacked at least some documentation of the reviews they told us they conducted, and in some cases, we found that the required reviews were not conducted at all. Specifically, across the five VA medical centers, we found the following:

- The medical centers lacked documentation showing that one type of review—focused professional practice evaluations (FPPE) for cause—had been conducted for 26 providers after concerns had been raised about their care. FPPEs for cause are reviews of providers' care over a specified period of time, during which the provider continues to see patients and has the opportunity to demonstrate improvement. Documentation of these reviews is explicitly required under VHA policy. Additionally, VA medical center officials confirmed that FPPEs for cause that were required for another 21 providers were never conducted.
- The medical centers lacked documentation showing that retrospective reviews—which assess the care previously delivered by a provider during a specific period of time— had been conducted for 8 providers after concerns had been raised about their clinical care.
- One medical center lacked documentation showing that reviews had been conducted for another 12 providers after concerns had been raised about their care. In the absence of any documentation,

we were unable to identify the types of reviews, if any, that were conducted for these 12 providers.

We also found that the five selected VA medical centers did not always conduct reviews of providers' clinical care in a timely manner. Specifically, of the 148 providers, the VA medical centers did not initiate reviews of 16 providers for 3 months, and in some cases, for multiple years, after concerns had been raised about the providers' care. In a few of these cases, additional concerns about the providers' clinical care were raised before the reviews began.

We found that two factors were largely responsible for the inadequate documentation and untimely reviews of providers' clinical care we identified at the selected VA medical centers.

- First, VHA policy does not require VA medical centers to document all types of reviews of providers' clinical care, including retrospective reviews, and VHA has not established a timeliness requirement for initiating reviews of providers' clinical care.
- Second, VHA's oversight of the reviews of providers' clinical care is inadequate. Under VHA policy, networks are responsible for overseeing the credentialing and privileging processes at their respective VA medical centers. While reviews of providers' clinical care after concerns are raised are a component of credentialing and privileging, we found that none of the network officials we spoke with described any routine oversight of such reviews.[6] This may be in part because the standardized tool that VHA requires the networks to use during their routine audits does not direct network officials to ensure that all reviews of providers' clinical care have been conducted and documented. Further, some

[6] When asked about their routine audits, network officials we interviewed generally described selecting a sample of providers from different specialties to review their compliance with VHA requirements related to credentialing and privileging. For example, network officials may check that medical centers have appropriately verified their providers' medical licensure. Some officials said they may also look at documentation of a VA medical center's review of a provider's clinical care after a concern had been raised if any of the providers in their sample happened to have documentation of such concerns in their files.

of the VISN officials we interviewed told us they were not using the standardized audit tool as required.

Without adequate documentation and timely completion of reviews of providers' clinical care, VA medical center officials lack the information they need to make decisions about providers' privileges, including whether or not to take adverse privileging actions against providers. Furthermore, because of its inadequate oversight, VHA lacks reasonable assurance that VA medical center officials are reviewing all providers about whom clinical care concerns have been raised and are taking adverse privileging actions against the providers when appropriate. To address these shortcomings, we recommended that VHA 1) require documentation of all reviews of providers' clinical care after concerns have been raised, 2) establish a timeliness requirement for initiating such reviews, and 3) strengthen its oversight by requiring networks to oversee VA medical centers to ensure that such reviews are documented and initiated in a timely manner. VA concurred with these recommendations and described plans for VHA to revise existing policy and update the standardized audit tool used by the networks to include more comprehensive oversight of VA medical centers' reviews of providers' clinical care after concerns have been raised.

SELECTED VA MEDICAL CENTERS DID NOT REPORT ALL PROVIDERS TO THE NPDB OR TO STATE LICENSING BOARDS AS REQUIRED

We found that from October 2013 through March 2017, the five VA medical centers we reviewed had only reported one of nine providers required to be reported to the NPDB under VHA policy. These nine providers either had adverse privileging actions taken against them or resigned or retired while under investigation before an adverse privileging action could be taken. None of these nine providers were reported to state licensing boards as required by VHA policy.

The VA medical centers documented that these nine providers had significant clinical deficiencies that sometimes resulted in adverse outcomes for veterans. For example, the documentation shows that one provider's surgical incompetence resulted in numerous repeat surgeries for veterans. Another provider's opportunity to improve through an FPPE for cause had to be halted and the provider was removed from providing care after only a week due to concerns that continuing the review would potentially harm patients.

In addition to these nine providers, one VA medical center terminated the services of four contract providers based on deficiencies in the providers' clinical performance, but the facility did not follow any of the required steps for reporting providers to the NPDB or relevant state licensing boards. This is concerning, given that the VA medical center documented that one of these providers was terminated for cause related to patient abuse after only 2 weeks of work at the facility.

Two of the five VA medical centers we reviewed each reported one provider to the state licensing boards for failing to meet generally accepted standards of clinical practice to the point that it raised concerns for the safety of veterans.[7] However, we found that the medical centers' reporting to the state licensing board took over 500 days to complete in both cases, which was significantly longer than the 100 days suggested in VHA policy.

Across the five VA medical centers, we found that providers were not reported to the NPDB and state licensing boards as required for two reasons.

- First, VA medical center officials were generally not familiar with or misinterpreted VHA policies related to NPDB and state licensing board reporting. For example, at one VA medical center, we found that officials failed to report six providers to the NPDB

---

[7] These two providers were not among the nine providers who had an adverse privileging action taken against them, resigned or retired while under investigation but before an adverse privileging action could be taken. They were also not among the four contractors whose services were terminated.

because they were unaware that they had been delegated responsibility for NPDB reporting.[8] Officials at two other VA medical centers incorrectly told us that VHA cannot report contract providers to the NDPB. At another VA medical facility, officials did not report a provider to the NPDB or to any of the state licensing boards where the provider held a medical license because medical center officials learned that one state licensing board had already found out about the issue independently. Therefore, VA officials did not believe that they needed to report the provider. This misinterpretation of VHA policy meant that the NPDB and the state licensing boards in other states where the provider held licenses were not alerted to concerns about the provider's clinical practice.

- Second, VHA policy does not require the networks to oversee whether VA medical centers are reporting providers to the NPDB or state licensing boards when warranted. We found, for example, that network officials were unaware of situations in which VA medical center officials failed to report providers to the NPDB. We concluded that VHA lacks reasonable assurance that all providers who should be reported to these entities are reported.

VHA's failure to report providers to the NPDB and state licensing boards as required facilitates providers who provide substandard care at one facility obtaining privileges at another VA medical center or at hospitals outside of VA's health care system. We found several cases of this occurring among the providers who were not reported to the NPDB or state licensing boards by the five VA medical centers we reviewed. For example, we found that two of the four contract providers whose contracts were terminated for clinical deficiencies remained eligible to provide care to veterans outside of that VA medical center. At the time of our review, one of these providers held privileges at another VA medical center, and

[8] As a result of our audit work, in August 2017, officials at this VA medical center reported three of these six providers to the NPDB.

another participated in the network of providers that can provide care for veterans in the community. We also found that a provider who was not reported as required to the NPDB during the period we reviewed had their privileges revoked 2 years later by a non-VA hospital in the same city for the same reason the provider was under investigation at the VA medical center. Officials at this VA medical center did not report this provider following a settlement agreement under which the provider agreed to resign. A committee within the VA medical center had recommended that the provider's privileges be revoked prior to the agreement. There was no documentation of the reasons why this provider was not reported to the NPDB under VHA policy.

To improve VA medical centers' reporting of providers to the NPDB and state licensing boards and VHA oversight of these processes, we recommended that VHA require its networks to establish a process for overseeing VA medical centers to ensure they are reporting to the NPDB and to state licensing boards and to ensure that this reporting is timely. VA concurred with this recommendation and told us that it plans to include oversight of timely reporting to the NPDB and state licensing boards as part of the standard audit tool used by the networks.

Chairman Bergman, Ranking Member Kuster, and Members of the Subcommittee, this concludes my statement. I would be pleased to respond to any questions that you may have at this time.

In: Improvements Needed in the VA … ISBN: 978-1-53615-971-4
Editor: Charles Copeland

Chapter 3

VA Health Care: Improvements Needed in Suicide Prevention Media Outreach Campaign Oversight and Evaluation*

United States Government Accountability Office

Abbreviations

CDC	Centers for Disease Control and Prevention
OMHSP	Office of Mental Health and Suicide Prevention
PSA	public service announcement
REACH VET	Recovery Engagement and Coordination for Health – Veterans Enhanced Treatment
VA	Department of Veterans Affairs
VCL	Veterans Crisis Line
VHA	Veterans Health Administration

* This is an edited, reformatted and augmented version of United States Government Accountability Office, Report to the Ranking Member Committee on Veterans' Affairs, House of Representatives, Publication No. GAO-19-66, dated November 2018.

Why GAO Did This Study

Veterans suffer a disproportionately higher rate of suicide than the civilian population. VA has estimated that an average of 20 veterans die by suicide per day, and in 2018, VA identified suicide prevention as its highest clinical priority. VHA's suicide prevention media outreach campaign—its collective suicide prevention outreach activities—helps raise awareness among veterans and others in the community about suicide prevention resources. VHA has contracted with an outside vendor to develop suicide prevention media outreach content.

GAO was asked to examine VHA's suicide prevention media outreach campaign. This chapter examines the extent to which VHA (1) conducts activities for its suicide prevention media outreach campaign, and (2) evaluates the effectiveness of its campaign. GAO reviewed relevant VHA documents and data on the amount, type, and cost of suicide prevention outreach activities since fiscal year 2013. GAO also reviewed VHA's contract for developing suicide prevention outreach content and interviewed VA and VHA officials.

What GAO Recommends

VHA should (1) establish an approach to oversee its suicide prevention media outreach campaign that includes clear delineation of roles and responsibilities, and (2) establish targets for its metrics to improve evaluation efforts. VA concurred with GAO's recommendations and described steps it will take to implement them.

What GAO Found

The Department of Veterans Affairs' (VA) Veterans Health Administration (VHA) conducts national suicide prevention media outreach on various platforms to raise awareness about VHA's suicide prevention resources. The primary focus of this campaign since 2010 has been to raise awareness of the Veterans Crisis Line (VCL), VHA's national hotline established in 2007 to provide support to veterans in emotional crisis. GAO found that VHA's suicide prevention media outreach activities declined in recent years due to leadership turnover and reorganization. For example, the amount of suicide prevention content developed by VHA's contractor for social media decreased in fiscal years 2017 and the first 10 months of 2018 after increasing in each of the 4 prior years.

VHA officials reported not having leadership available for a period of time to make decisions about the suicide prevention media outreach campaign. GAO found that VHA did not assign key leadership responsibilities or establish clear lines of reporting, and as a result, its ability to oversee the outreach campaign was hindered. Consequently, VHA may not be maximizing its reach with suicide prevention media content to veterans, especially those who are at-risk.

VHA evaluates the effectiveness of its suicide prevention media outreach campaign by collecting data on metrics, such as the number of people that visit the VCL website. However, VHA has not established targets for the majority of these metrics. Officials said they have not established targets because, apart from one industry-wide target they use, they lack meaningful targets for evaluating the campaign. However, VHA could use information about how its metrics performed in the past to develop reasonable and meaningful targets for future performance. Without established targets for its metrics, VHA is missing an opportunity to better evaluate the effectiveness of its suicide prevention media outreach campaign.

November 15, 2018

The Honorable Tim Walz
Ranking Member
Committee on Veterans' Affairs
House of Representatives

Dear Mr. Walz:

Suicide is a public health problem facing all populations, particularly veterans. After military service, veterans suffer a disproportionately higher rate of suicide than the civilian population. According to the Department of Veterans Affairs (VA), veterans accounted for 14.3 percent of all deaths by suicide among United States adults in 2015, despite constituting only 8.3 percent of the adult population. VA reported in June 2018 that an average of 20 veterans died by suicide each day in 2015, and that an average of 6 of these 20 veterans (30 percent) were recent users of VA's Veterans Health Administration's (VHA) health care services.[1] Suicide is not unique to veterans; the Centers for Disease Control and Prevention (CDC) reports that suicide was the tenth leading cause of death in the United States in 2015.[2] However, according to VA, the rate of suicide is higher for veterans than non-veterans (see Figure 1).

VHA conducts national outreach to veterans and others in the community to raise awareness about suicide prevention and services available through VA, as one of several VHA initiatives to help reduce suicides in the veteran community. Since 2010, VHA has awarded multiple contracts to the same vendor to develop content for suicide prevention media outreach.[3] Questions have been raised about the effectiveness of VHA's collective suicide prevention media outreach activities, also referred to as its suicide prevention media outreach campaign. You asked us to review VHA's suicide prevention media outreach activities and related oversight. In this chapter, we examine:

1. the extent to which VHA conducts activities for its suicide prevention media outreach campaign; and

---

[1] See Department of Veterans Affairs, *VA National Suicide Data Report* (Washington, D.C.: June 2018). VA's June 2018 report is based on 2015 data, the most recent year of data available. Recent users of VHA health care services is defined as those who received VHA care in 2015 or 2014.

[2] See Centers for Disease Control and Prevention, *Preventing Suicide: A Technical Package of Policy, Programs, and Practices* (Atlanta, Ga.: 2017).

[3] Outreach "content" refers to materials for communicating with the public, such as flyers, and billboards, and social media posts. VHA's suicide prevention content typically includes images and information about its suicide prevention services and resources.

2. the extent to which VHA evaluates the effectiveness of its suicide prevention media outreach campaign.

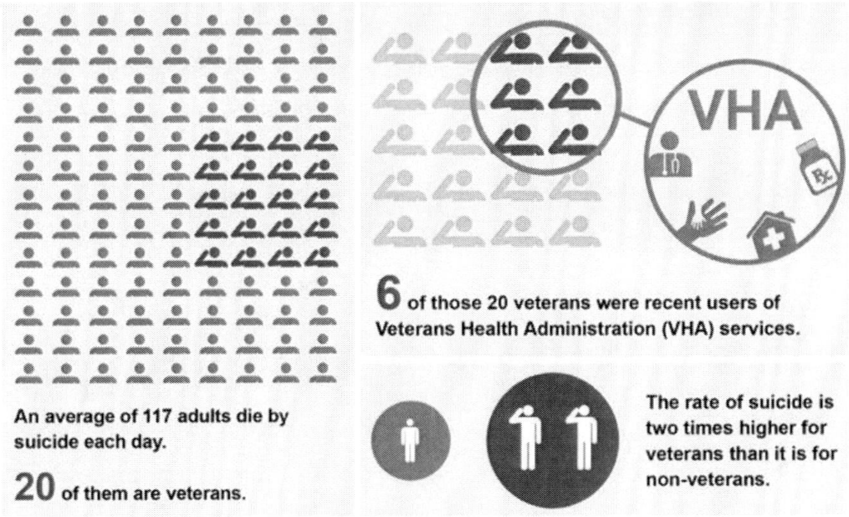

Source: Department of Veterans Affairs (VA). | GAO-19-66.

Note: See Department of Veterans Affairs, *VA National Suicide Data Report* (Washington, D.C.: June 2018). The report includes data from 2015, the most recent year of complete data available. In its agency comments, VA indicated that the rate of suicide is now one and a half times higher for veterans than it is for non-veterans, based on its September 2018 report, which includes data through 2016. See VA, *VA National Suicide Data Report* (Washington, D.C.: September 2018).

Figure 1. Veteran Suicide Rates Compared to Non-Veterans, 2015.

To examine the extent to which VHA conducts activities for its suicide prevention media outreach campaign, we reviewed VHA's contract to develop suicide prevention outreach content from fiscal years 2013 through 2016 and its contract to develop suicide prevention and mental health outreach content in fiscal years 2017 and 2018.[5] VHA's first such contract began in 2010; however, the Federal Acquisition Regulation only requires federal agencies to maintain contract documentation for a period

[5] Both contracts are with the same vendor, which we will refer to hereafter as VHA's "contractor."

of 6 years after the last payment. Therefore, we did not include the initial contract or associated outreach in our review due to the lack of available documentation. We also requested and reviewed data on the amount and type of outreach content that VHA's contractor developed from fiscal year 2013 through fiscal year 2018.[6] We interviewed VHA officials responsible for implementation and oversight of the contract about the data. We also obtained written responses from the contractor about the steps it took to compile and ensure the accuracy of the data. On the basis of these actions, we found these data to be sufficiently reliable for the purpose of our reporting objective.

We also reviewed documentation and interviewed VHA officials who worked on the campaign about VHA's suicide prevention media outreach campaign, outreach activities, and VHA leadership officials' involvement in the campaign, and plans moving forward.[7] We compared VHA's outreach campaign and related activities with federal internal control standards related to control environment and monitoring.[8] We also interviewed relevant other VHA and VA officials who played a role in the suicide prevention media outreach campaign, including officials in VA's Office of Acquisitions, Logistics, and Construction and VHA's Office of Communications.

To examine the extent to which VHA evaluates the effectiveness of its suicide prevention media outreach campaign, we reviewed documentation of VHA's evaluation efforts, including monthly monitoring reports, to identify any performance metrics VHA monitors and any targets

---

[6] In order to expedite this data request, VHA enlisted the assistance of the contractor to provide the data in the format and time frames required for this review. We requested the data on a subset of the types of content the contractor develops in order to focus on those types of media outreach most relevant to our work. For example, we did not focus on promotional items, such as magnets and keychains, and data on website maintenance. For fiscal year 2018, we obtained data through July 2018, the first 10 months of the fiscal year.

[7] Officials that worked on the campaign include the contracting officer's representative (the primary VHA official responsible for oversight of the contract) and other officials within VHA that worked directly on the campaign.

[8] GAO, *Standards for Internal Control in the Federal Government*, GAO-14-704G (Washington, D.C.: Sept. 10, 2014) and *Standards for Internal Control in the Federal Government*, GAO/AIMD-00-21.3.1 (Washington, D.C.: Nov. 1, 1999). Internal control is a process effected by an entity's management, oversight body, and other personnel that provides reasonable assurance that the objectives of an entity will be achieved.

established for those metrics. We also reviewed the 2016 contract to identify any requirements for the contractor to monitor and report on the effectiveness of the campaign. Additionally, we interviewed VHA officials responsible for monitoring and evaluating the campaign and reviewed supporting documentation. Specifically, we asked officials about the extent to which they had evaluated the campaign's effectiveness since fiscal year 2013, their evaluation processes and tools, and any plans for completing future evaluations. We then compared VHA's evaluation efforts to criteria we developed in previous bodies of work for designing program evaluations, as well as to federal internal control standards for monitoring.[9]

We conducted this performance audit from December 2017 to November 2018 in accordance with generally accepted government auditing standards. Those standards require that we plan and perform the audit to obtain sufficient, appropriate evidence to provide a reasonable basis for our findings and conclusions based on our audit objectives. We believe that the evidence obtained provides a reasonable basis for our findings and conclusions based on our audit objectives.

BACKGROUND

VA Suicide Prevention

VA has undertaken a number of initiatives to help prevent veteran suicide, including identifying suicide prevention as VA's highest clinical priority in its strategic plan for fiscal years 2018 through 2024 (see Figure 2).[10]

[9] GAO, *Tax Administration: IRS Needs to Further Refine Its Tax Filing Season Performance Measures*, GAO-03-143 (Washington, D.C.: Nov. 22, 2002). Our prior work states that clearly articulating a program's strategy and performance expectations aids the selection of appropriate performance measures and data sources. For example, a well-articulated program logic model can help evaluate agency efforts. See also GAO, *Designing Evaluations: 2012 Revision,* GAO-12-208G (Washington, D.C.: Jan. 31, 2012), GAO-14-704G, and GAO/AIMD-00-21.3.1.

[10] See Department of Veterans Affairs, *Department of Veterans Affairs Fiscal Years 2018- 2024 Strategic Plan* (Washington, D.C.: Feb. 12, 2018).

VA uses CDC's research on risk factors and prevention techniques to inform its approach to suicide prevention in the veteran community. There is no single determining cause for suicide; instead, suicide occurs in response to biological, psychological, interpersonal, environmental, and societal influences, according to the CDC. Specifically, suicide is associated with risk factors that exist at the individual level (such as a history of mental illness or substance abuse, or stressful life events, such as divorce or the death of a loved one), community level (such as barriers to health care), or societal level (such as the way suicide is portrayed in the media and stigma associated with seeking help for mental illness).

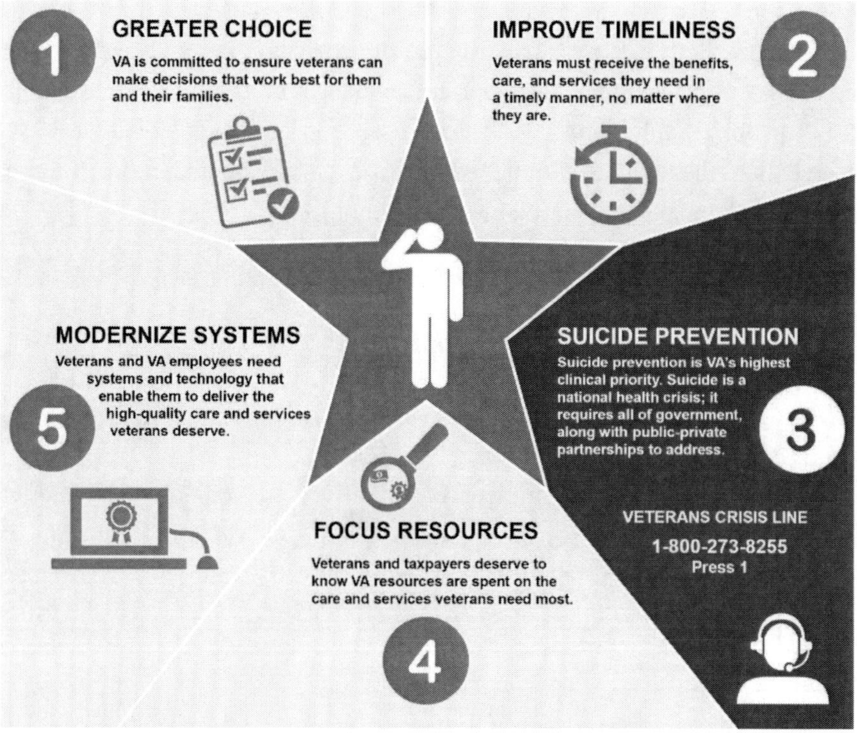

Source: VA (information); GAO (illustration). | GAO-19-66.

Figure 2. Top Five Priorities in the Department of Veterans Affairs' (VA) Strategic Plan for Fiscal Years 2018–2024.

According to VA, veterans may possess risk factors related to their military service, such as a service-related injury or a difficult transition to civilian life. CDC reports that protective factors—influences that help protect against the risk for suicide—include effective coping and problem-solving skills, strong and supportive relationships with friends and family, availability of health care, and connectedness to social institutions such as school and community. VA's 2018 National Strategy for Suicide Prevention identifies four focus areas: (1) healthy and empowered veterans, families, and communities; (2) clinical and community preventative services; (3) treatment and support services; and (4) surveillance, research, and evaluation.[11] Collectively, these four areas encompass 14 goals for preventing veteran suicide, one of which is implementing communication designed to prevent veteran suicide by changing knowledge, attitude, and behaviors.

VHA's suicide prevention media outreach campaign is just one of its initiatives intended to reduce veteran suicide. For example, in 2007, VHA established the Veteran's Crisis Line (VCL), a national toll-free hotline that supports veterans in emotional crisis.[12] Veterans, as well as their family and friends, can access the VCL by calling a national toll-free number—1-800-273-8255—and pressing "1" to be connected with a VCL responder, regardless of whether these veterans receive health care through VHA. VHA added the option to communicate with VCL responders via online chat in 2009, followed by text messaging in 2011. Another VHA suicide prevention initiative is the Recovery Engagement and Coordination for Health – Veterans Enhanced Treatment initiative, or REACH VET. Established in 2016, REACH VET uses predictive modeling to analyze

---

[11] Department of Veterans Affairs, *National Strategy for Preventing Veteran Suicide 2018- 2028* (Washington, D.C.: June 29, 2018).

[12] We have previously reported on the VCL and made recommendations for improving the timeliness and quality of VA's VCL responses. VA concurred with our recommendations and in July 2016, developed and implemented procedures to regularly test the VCL system. In addition, in July 2017, VA updated its VCL quality assurance plan to document measurable targets and time frames for key performance indicators needed to assess the VCL's performance. See GAO, *Veterans Crisis Line: Additional Testing, Monitoring, and Information Needed to Ensure Better Quality Service,* GAO-16-373 (Washington, D.C.: May 26, 2016).

existing data from veterans' health records to identify veterans at increased risk for adverse outcomes, such as suicide, hospitalization, or illness.[13]

VHA's Suicide Prevention Media Outreach Campaign

Suicide prevention officials within VHA's Office of Mental Health and Suicide Prevention (OMHSP) are responsible for implementing the suicide prevention media outreach campaign. Since 2010, VHA has used a contractor to develop suicide prevention media outreach content and monitor its effectiveness. In September 2016, VHA awarded a new contract to the same contractor to provide both suicide prevention and mental health media outreach. Under the 2016 contract, the suicide prevention and mental health outreach campaigns remain separate and are overseen by separate suicide prevention and mental health officials, both within OMHSP.[14] VHA officials told us that beginning in fiscal year 2019, VHA will separate the contract for suicide prevention and mental health media outreach. Specifically, VHA will utilize an existing agreement with a different contractor for suicide prevention media outreach while the existing contractor will continue to provide mental health media outreach.[15]

According to VHA, the purpose of its suicide prevention media outreach campaign is to raise awareness among veterans, their families and friends, and the general public about VHA resources that are available to veterans who may be at risk for suicide.

---

[13] After being identified by REACH VET, veterans are contacted by VA health care providers to determine whether additional care or services are needed.

[14] VHA officials said OMHSP was established in May 2017. Before May 2017, the suicide prevention program and the mental health program were organizationally located under different offices within VHA. In addition to these two programs, OMHSP also includes the VCL program, among others.

[15] Specifically, VHA said it will utilize an existing blanket purchase agreement through a GSA schedule contract. A blanket purchase agreement is a simplified method of filling anticipated repetitive needs for supplies or services that functions as a charge account, with terms and conditions agreed upon when the blanket purchase agreement is established. Federal Acquisition Regulation §§ 8.405-3, 13.303-1(a).

The primary focus of the outreach campaign since 2010 has been to raise awareness of the services available through the VCL.[16]

VHA's suicide prevention media outreach falls into two main categories: unpaid and paid. Unpaid media outreach content is typically displayed on platforms owned by VA or VHA, or is disseminated by external organizations or individuals that share VHA suicide prevention content at no cost, as discussed below (see Figure 3).[17]

- Social media. VA and VHA each maintain national social media accounts on platforms such as Facebook, Twitter, and Instagram, and post content, including suicide prevention content developed by VHA's contractor.[18] VHA also works with other federal agencies, non-governmental organizations, and individuals that post its suicide prevention content periodically.
- Public service announcements (PSA). VHA's contractor typically develops two PSAs per year, which various local and national media networks display at no cost to VHA.
- Website. VHA's contractor maintains the content displayed on the VCL website (veteranscrisisline.net), including much of the content it develops for other platforms, such as PSAs and social media content. Visitors to the website can both view the content on the website and share it on their own platforms.

Paid media outreach includes outreach on media platforms for which VHA must pay a fee to display its content (see Figure 4). Paid media falls into two categories, as discussed below.

---

[16] See GAO-16-373.

[17] VHA also conducts unpaid outreach in the form of attending conferences and seminars, as well as developing materials to hand out to veterans and the community at these and other events. However, this type of outreach was not the focus of our report because it is not a national, media-based outreach effort.

[18] VHA has a VCL Facebook page, but officials told us that they intentionally do not populate it with suicide prevention content because it would not be an appropriate resource for providing timely support to veterans in emotional crisis.

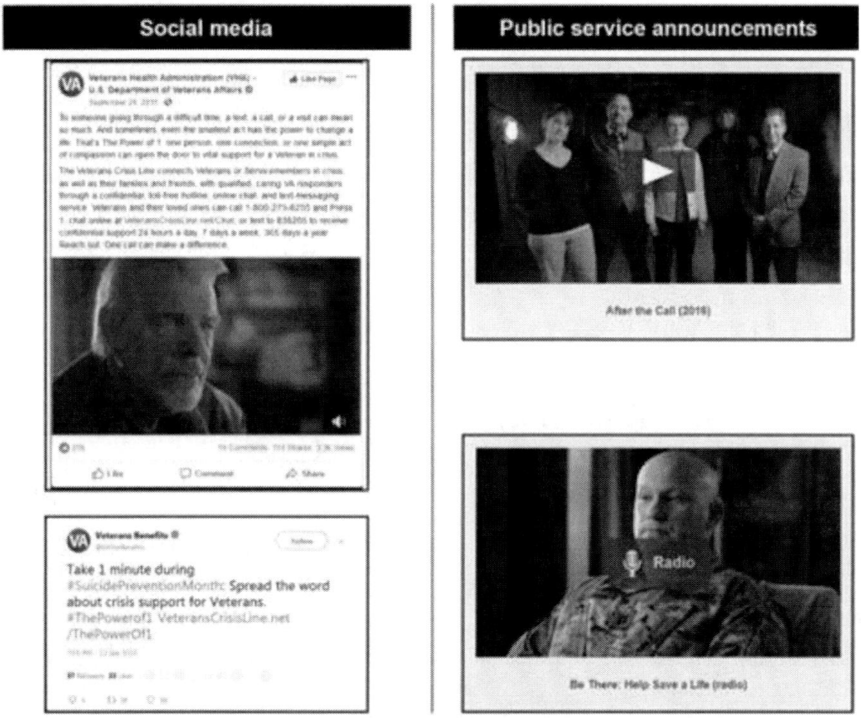

Source: © J.R. Reingold & Associates, Inc. | GAO-19-66.

Note: Unpaid media refers to outreach content that is displayed on platforms owned by the Department of Veterans Affairs, or is disseminated by external organizations or individuals that share VHA suicide prevention content at no cost.

Figure 3. Examples of the Veterans Health Administration's (VHA) Unpaid Suicide Prevention Media Outreach Content.

- Paid digital media. An example of paid digital media includes online keyword searches, in which VHA pays a search engine a fee for its website to appear as a top result in response to selected keywords, such as "veterans crisis line" or "veteran suicide." Paid digital media also includes social media posts for which VHA pays a fee to display its content to a widespread audience, such as users with a military affiliation.
- Paid "out-of-home" media: "Out-of-home" refers to the locations where this type of content is typically displayed. Examples include

billboards, bus and transit advertisements, and local and national radio commercials.

VHA recognizes September as Suicide Prevention Month each year. During this month, VHA establishes a theme and increases its outreach activities, including a combination of both paid and unpaid media outreach. According to VHA, it typically incorporates additional outreach techniques during this month, such as enlisting the support of celebrities or hosting live chat sessions on social media platforms, including Facebook and Twitter.

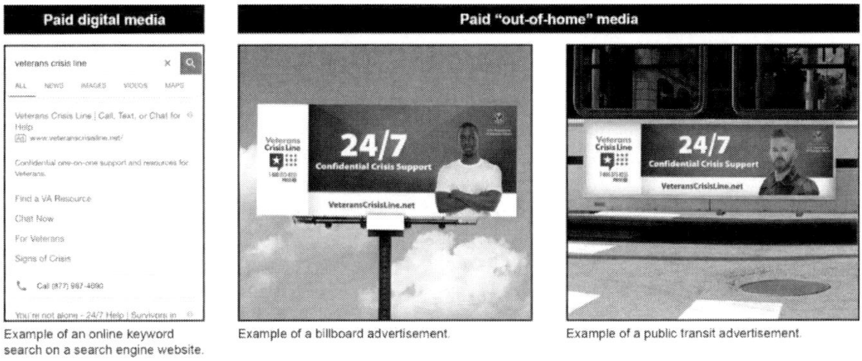

Source: © J.R. Reingold & Associates, Inc. | GAO-19-66.

Figure 4. Examples of the Veterans Health Administration's Paid Suicide Prevention Media Outreach Content.

VHA's Suicide Prevention Media Outreach Activities Declined in Recent Years Due to Leadership Turnover and Reorganization

VHA's Suicide Prevention Media Outreach Activities Declined in Fiscal Years 2017 and 2018

VHA's suicide prevention media outreach activities declined in fiscal years 2017 and 2018 compared to earlier years of the campaign. We identified declines in social media postings, PSAs, paid media, and suicide prevention month activities, as discussed below.

- Social media. The amount of social media content developed by VHA's contractor decreased in 2017 and 2018, after increasing in each of the prior four years. Specifically, VHA reported that its contractor developed 339 pieces of social media content in fiscal year 2016, compared with 159 in fiscal year 2017, and 47 during the first 10 months of fiscal year 2018 (see Figure 5).[19]

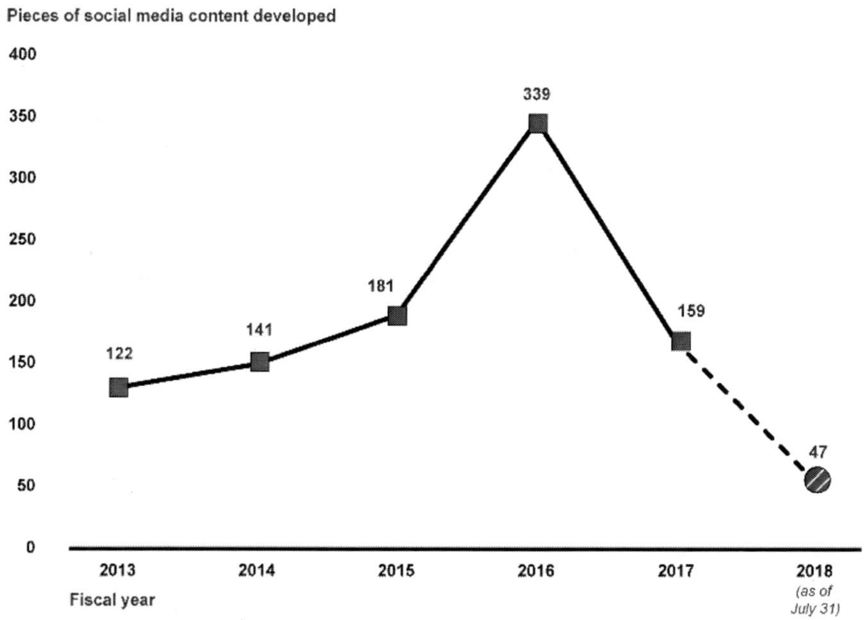

Source: Veterans Health Administration. | GAO-19-66.

Note: The table includes the amount of social media content developed, not the number of times it was posted on social media platforms or displayed in other locations.

Figure 5. Suicide Prevention Outreach Social Media Content Developed for the Veterans Health Administration, October 2012 through July 2018.

---

[19] The data includes the amount of content that was developed, not the number of times it was posted or displayed. This is because the outreach content developed by VHA's contractor is often disseminated on platforms that are not owned by VHA or its contractor.

- PSAs. VHA's contractor is required to develop two suicide prevention PSAs in each fiscal year. VHA officials said that the development of the two PSAs was delayed in fiscal year 2018. Specifically, as of August 2018, VHA reported that one PSA was completed, but had not yet aired, and another PSA was in development.[20] As a result of this delay, VHA had not aired a suicide prevention PSA on television or radio in over a year; this is the first time there has been a gap of more than a month since June 2012.
- Paid media. VHA had a total budget of $17.7 million for its suicide prevention and mental health media outreach for fiscal year 2018, of which $6.2 million was obligated for suicide prevention paid media. As of September 2018, VHA said it had spent $57,000 of its $6.2 million paid media budget.[21] VHA officials estimated that they would spend a total of $1.5 million on suicide prevention paid media for fiscal year 2018 and indicated that the remaining funds would be de-obligated from the contract at the end of the fiscal year and not used for suicide prevention media outreach. VHA officials indicated that the reason they did not spend the remaining funds on suicide prevention paid media in fiscal year 2018 was that the approval of the paid media plan was delayed due to changes in leadership and organizational realignment of the suicide prevention program. As a result, VHA officials said they limited the paid media outreach in fiscal year 2018 to activities that were already in place, including 25 keyword search advertisements, and 20 billboards and 8 radio advertisements in selected cities across the United States.

---

[20] VHA released a PSA on suicide prevention in October 2017. However, VHA officials said this PSA was not developed by the contractor, but through a partnership with an outside organization, and it was developed for online dissemination, as opposed to television or radio.

[21] VHA officials told us that because paid media is very effective, the amount of approved funds would be the biggest factor in determining the amount and type of paid media to conduct each year.

In prior fiscal years, VHA conducted a variety of digital and out-of-home suicide prevention paid media. For example, in fiscal year 2015, with a suicide prevention paid media budget of more than $4 million, VHA reported that it ran 58 advertisements on Google, Bing, and Facebook, and ran 30 billboards, 180 bus advertisements, more than 19,000 radio advertisements, 252 print advertisements, and 39 movie theatre placements in selected cities across the United States.[22] VHA ran similar types of paid media in fiscal years 2013, 2014, and 2016 with variation in quantities based on the approved budget in each of these years. In fiscal year 2017, VHA had a budget of approximately $1.7 million to spend on paid media for both the suicide prevention and mental health outreach campaigns. However, VHA spent less than 10 percent of the funds (approximately $136,000) to run paid advertisements on Google and Bing for suicide prevention in fiscal year 2017; the remainder was spent on mental health outreach.

- Suicide Prevention Month. VHA documentation indicated that Suicide Prevention Month 2017 was a limited effort. VHA officials said that this was because they did not begin preparing early enough. In May 2018, VHA officials indicated that they were similarly behind schedule for planning Suicide Prevention Month 2018, though they told us in August 2018 that they had caught up.

VHA Leadership Turnover and Reorganization Resulted in the Decline in Suicide Prevention Media Outreach Activities

VHA officials told us that the decrease in suicide prevention media outreach activities was due to leadership turnover and reorganization since 2017. For example, VHA officials said the National Director for Suicide Prevention position was vacant from July 2017 through April 2018. VHA filled the role temporarily with a 6-month detail from another agency from

[22] In fiscal years 2014, 2015, and 2016, VHA paid movie theatres to show suicide prevention PSAs during the previews.

October 2017 through March 2018 and then hired this individual as the permanent director on April 30, 2018. VHA officials that worked on the campaign told us they did not have leadership available to make decisions about the suicide prevention campaign during this time. For example, VHA officials said they did not have a kick-off meeting between VHA leadership and VHA's contractor at the beginning of fiscal year 2018—a requirement of the contract—because there was no leadership available to participate in this meeting.[23]

The officials also reported that suicide prevention leadership was not available for weekly meetings to discuss suicide prevention outreach activities, even after the suicide prevention program obtained an acting director on detail from another agency. VHA staff said that at that time, they focused their suicide prevention media outreach efforts on areas that did not require leadership input, such as updating the VCL website. The absence of leadership available to provide direction and make decisions on the suicide prevention media outreach campaign is inconsistent with federal internal control standards for control environment, which require agencies to assign responsibilities to achieve its objectives.[24] If a key role is vacant, management needs to determine by whom and how those responsibilities will be fulfilled in order to meet its objectives.

Officials that worked on the campaign told us they shifted their focus away from the suicide prevention media outreach campaign toward the mental health outreach campaign due to reorganization of the offices responsible for suicide prevention activities in 2017. Specifically, under the new organization, and in the absence of suicide prevention program leadership, the officials began reporting directly to mental health program leadership and became more focused on the mental health outreach aspects of the contract.[25] Following the reorganization, officials that worked on the campaign did not have a clear line of reporting to the suicide prevention

[23] During kick-off meetings, VHA and its contractor typically discuss lessons learned from the prior year's campaign and the approach for the coming year, such as target audiences, outreach platforms, paid media, and new initiatives.

[24] GAO-14-704G and GAO/AIMD-00-21.3.1.

[25] VHA officials said that they had planned to appoint new staff to work specifically on the suicide prevention outreach campaign, but they had difficulty doing so until March 2018.

program. This is also inconsistent with federal internal control standards for control environment, which require agencies to establish an organizational structure and assign responsibilities, such as establishing lines of reporting necessary information to management.[26]

VHA officials told us that one of the highest priorities for the suicide prevention program since the beginning of fiscal year 2018 was to establish a national strategy for preventing veteran suicides. The national strategy, issued in June 2018, includes suicide prevention outreach as one of the strategy's 14 goals.[27] The national strategy also emphasizes VHA's plans to shift to a public health approach to suicide prevention outreach. The public health approach focuses less on raising awareness of the VCL and more on reaching veterans before the point of crisis.[28] VHA officials told us they have been trying to shift to a public health approach since 2016. Some of the campaign themes and messages have reflected this shift; for example, the "Be There" campaign theme that was adopted in fiscal year 2016—and has remained the theme since— emphasizes the message that everyone has a role in helping veterans in crisis feel less alone and connecting them to resources. However, VHA officials told us in May 2018 that they were just beginning to conceptualize what the suicide prevention outreach campaign should look like moving forward. Leadership officials also said that while they were developing the national strategy, they delegated the responsibility for implementing the suicide prevention outreach campaign to other officials working on the campaign.

The decline in VHA's suicide prevention media outreach activities over the past 2 fiscal years is inconsistent with VA's strategic goals, which identify suicide prevention as the agency's top clinical priority for fiscal years 2018 through 2024.[29] Further, VHA has continued to obligate millions of dollars to its suicide prevention media outreach campaign each year. Since fiscal year 2017, VHA has obligated $24.6 million to the

---

[26] GAO-14-704G and GAO/AIMD-00-21.3.1.

[27] VA, *National Strategy for Preventing Veteran Suicide 2018-2028.*

[28] Some VHA officials indicated that the shift away from raising awareness of the VCL was driven in part by reports that the VCL volume had exceeded its capacity for a period of time. However, VHA leadership officials, including the Director of the VCL, said that raising awareness of the VCL continues to be a priority.

[29] VA, *Department of Veterans Affairs Fiscal Years 2018- 2024 Strategic Plan.*

contract for media outreach related to both suicide prevention and mental health.[30]

By not assigning key leadership responsibilities and clear lines of reporting, VHA's ability to oversee the suicide prevention media outreach activities was hindered and these outreach activities decreased. As a result, VHA may not have exposed as many people in the community, such as veterans at risk for suicide, or their families and friends, to its suicide prevention outreach content. Additionally, without establishing responsibility and clear lines of reporting, VHA lacks assurance that it will have continuous oversight of its suicide prevention media outreach activities in the event of additional turnover and reorganization in the future, particularly as VHA begins implementing the suicide prevention media outreach campaign under its new agreement that begins in fiscal year 2019.

VHA Monitors Metrics for Its Suicide Prevention Media Outreach Campaign, But Has Not Established Targets against Which to Evaluate the Campaign's Effectiveness

VHA Monitors Metrics for Its Suicide Prevention Media Outreach Campaign

VHA works with its contractor to create and monitor metrics to help gauge the effectiveness of its suicide prevention media outreach campaign in raising awareness among veterans and others about VHA services, such as the VCL. The metrics primarily focus on the number of individuals who were exposed to or interacted with VHA's suicide prevention content across various forms of outreach, including social media, PSAs, and

---

[30] Some of the deliverables in the fiscal year 2017 contract apply only to one campaign, while other deliverables are divided evenly between the two campaigns. Between fiscal years 2013 and 2016, VHA obligated over $16.8 million to the contract specifically for suicide prevention media outreach. These amounts include the cost of paid and unpaid media outreach, as well as indirect costs.

websites.[31] According to VHA, the metrics are intended to help VHA ensure that its media outreach activities achieve intended results, such as increasing awareness and use of the resources identified on the VCL website.[32] Examples of metrics monitored by VHA and its contractor include those related to (1) social media, such as the number of times a piece of outreach content is displayed on social media; (2) PSAs, such as the total number of markets and television stations airing a PSA; and (3) the VCL website, such as the total traffic to the website, as well as the average amount of time spent on a page and average number of pages viewed per visit. VHA's contractor is required to monitor the metrics and report results on a monthly basis. Specifically, the contractor provides monthly monitoring reports to VHA that summarize how outreach is performing, such as the number of visits to the VCL website that were driven from paid media sources. Officials noted these reports are key sources of information for VHA on the results of its outreach. VHA officials also told us they informally discuss certain metrics during weekly meetings with VHA's contractor. In addition, VHA works with its contractor to conduct a more in-depth analysis of outreach efforts during and after Suicide Prevention Month each year.

VHA Lacks Metric Targets to Evaluate the Effectiveness of Its Suicide Prevention Media Outreach Campaign

VHA has not established targets for the majority of the metrics it uses to help gauge the effectiveness of its suicide prevention media outreach

---

[31] Specifically, for its suicide prevention media outreach, VHA tracks reach, impressions and engagement. For the purposes of this report, "reach" refers to the number of unique people who may have seen a piece of outreach content, while "impressions" typically estimate the total number of times a piece of outreach content was displayed to people. For example, if VHA posts two tweets and 100 people see both of them, the reach is 100 while the impressions are 200. Meanwhile, "engagement" typically measures the number of times the audience interacted with a piece of outreach content, including click-through rates (the percentage of people exposed to an advertisement who click on it to access the advertised website) and social media "likes." These metrics can help VHA gauge the extent to which its outreach is raising awareness of the VCL and other VHA services through its outreach.

[32] VHA officials acknowledged that some metric outcomes can be affected by events or factors outside of VHA's control. For example, certain public events can raise awareness of suicide risk and increase calls to the VCL or visits to the VCL website.

campaign. As a result, VHA does not have the information it needs to fully evaluate the campaign's effectiveness in raising awareness of VHA's suicide prevention resources among veterans, including the VCL.[33] For example, we found that VHA's contractor's monitoring reports—a summary of key metrics that VHA uses to routinely monitor information regarding the campaign—generally focused on outreach "highlights" and positive results. The reports did not set expectations based on past outreach or targets for new outreach, and lacked more comprehensive information on whether outreach performed against these expectations. For example:

- A monitoring report from 2018 showed that during one month, there were 21,000 social media mentions of keywords specific to VA suicide prevention, such as "VCL" or "veteran suicide," across social media platforms. These mentions earned 120 million impressions; however, there was no indication of the number of keyword mentions or impressions that VHA expected based on its media outreach activities. In addition, the report did not indicate the proportion of mentions that VHA believed were specifically driven by its outreach activities, and there also was no indication of whether these mentions were positive or negative, or what actions to take based on this information.[34]
- Another monitoring report from January 2017 showed that paid advertising drove 39 percent of overall website traffic during one month, while unpaid sources drove the remaining 61 percent. However, there was no information indicating the amounts of paid advertising that VHA conducted during this monitoring period,

[33] While VHA has not established targets for the majority of its metrics, we found that VHA had established one specific target for its suicide prevention PSAs. Specifically, VHA officials told us their goal for each PSA is to rank in the top 10 percent of the Nielsen ratings; VHA's contractor tracks these metrics and provides feedback to VHA through PSA monitoring reports. Nielsen ratings are a tool used to measure audience television viewership and are produced by The Nielsen Company (U.S.), LLC, a data analytics company.

[34] The social media mentions metric can capture negative publicity about VHA or the VCL. For example, it could include Instagram or Facebook posts about unsatisfactory experiences with the VCL, such as long wait times

and whether this amount of website traffic from paid advertising met expectations.

- VHA's 2016 Suicide Prevention Month summary report showed that there were 194,536 visits to the VCL website, roughly an 8 percent increase from the Suicide Prevention Month in 2015. However, the report did not indicate whether this increase from the prior year met expectations, or a different result was expected.

VHA officials told us that they have not established targets for most of the suicide prevention media outreach campaign because they lack meaningful targets for the metrics to help evaluate the campaign. VHA officials said that the only target they have established is for each PSA to rank in the top 10 percent of the Nielsen ratings because this is the only meaningful target available that is accepted industry-wide.[35] VHA officials stated that using any other targets would be arbitrary. For the remaining metrics, VHA officials told us they assess the outcomes of their campaign by comparing data from year to year, and examining any changes in the outcomes over time.[36] However, VHA could set targets that capture the

---

[35] Apart from noting the lack of meaningful targets for their metrics, officials also noted that it is generally difficult to determine whether behavioral shifts have occurred in veterans as a result of VA's outreach efforts and that they have struggled to study these types of outcomes. For example, in 2017, OMHSP proposed collaborating with VA's Center of Excellence for Suicide Prevention, whose mission is in part to use research to inform the implementation of effective veteran suicide prevention strategies, to (1) examine the metrics for the suicide prevention media outreach campaign, and (2) obtain veterans perspectives on the campaign. However, officials said that this effort did not commence due to the lack of senior leadership during and after this time. Officials indicated they would like to continue with their evaluation efforts in the future. VA's Center of Excellence has completed other studies that have examined the effects of VA's suicide prevention campaign. For example, one study that examined associations between VA's suicide prevention campaign and the use of crisis support services found that there were significant increases in call volume to the VCL to both targeted and broad resources during the campaign. See Elizabeth Karras, Naiji Lus, Guoxin Zuo, Xin M. Tu, Brady Stephens, John Draper, Caitlin Thompson, and Robert M. Bossarte, "Measuring Associations of the Department of Veterans Affairs' Suicide Prevention Campaign on the Use of Crisis Support Services," *Suicide and Life-Threatening Behavior,* 46 (4) August 2016: 447-456.

[36] VHA officials shared that their general approach has been to improve their suicide prevention media outreach activities each year by increasing the number of materials issued and website visits because, officials said, this means more people are being reached. They said that the indirect result of reaching more people is that the number of VCL calls are increasing, meaning more people are aware of VA's outreach activities. However, officials also recognized the number of visits to the website will likely reach a maximum after a

number of people who viewed or interacted with its outreach content, similar to its Nielsen target set for television viewership. Doing so would help VHA evaluate whether the campaign has been effective in raising awareness of VHA's suicide prevention resources. Further, creating targets for these additional metrics need not be arbitrary, because VHA could use information about how its metrics performed in the past to develop reasonable and meaningful targets for future performance. VHA could also adjust the targets over time to reflect changes in its metrics or approach to the campaign, such as changes to its paid media budget each year.

Federal internal control standards for monitoring require agencies to assess the quality of its performance by evaluating the results of activities. Agencies can then use these evaluations to determine the effectiveness of its programs or need for any corrective actions.[37] Further, VA's June 2018 National Strategy for Preventing Veteran Suicide also emphasizes the importance of the agency evaluating the effectiveness of its outreach.[38] The absence of established targets leaves VHA without a framework to effectively evaluate its campaign. Our prior work has shown that establishing targets allows agencies to track their progress toward specific goals. In particular, we have developed several key attributes of performance goals and measures including, when appropriate, the development of quantifiable, numerical targets for performance goals and measures.[39] Such targets can facilitate future evaluations of whether overall goals and objectives were achieved by allowing for comparisons between projected performance and actual results. Further, establishing targets for its outreach metrics will enable VHA officials to determine whether outreach performed as expected and raised awareness of VHA resources such as the VCL, including identifying outreach efforts that worked particularly well and those that did not. In doing so, VHA officials will have the opportunity to make better informed decisions in their suicide

certain point, and their goal might shift to maintaining the number of website visits rather than increasing it.

[37] GAO-14-704G and GAO/AIMD-00-21.3.1.

[38] VA, *National Strategy for Preventing Veteran Suicide 2012-2018*.

[39] GAO-03-143 and GAO-12-208G.

prevention media outreach campaign to support VA's overall goal of reducing veteran suicides.

CONCLUSION

VA has stated that preventing veteran suicide is its top clinical priority; yet VHA's lack of leadership attention to its suicide prevention media outreach campaign in recent years has resulted in less outreach to veterans. While VHA identifies the campaign as its primary method of raising suicide prevention awareness, it has not established an effective oversight approach to ensure outreach continuity. This became particularly evident during a recent period of turnover and reorganization in the office responsible for the suicide prevention outreach campaign. Moving forward, VHA has an opportunity to improve its oversight to ensure that its outreach content reaches veterans and others in the community to raise awareness of VHA's suicide prevention services, particularly as VHA begins working with a new contractor beginning in fiscal year 2019. VHA is responsible for evaluating the effectiveness of its suicide prevention media outreach campaign in raising awareness about VHA services that are available to veterans who may be at risk for suicide. To do so, VHA collects and monitors data on campaign metrics to help gauge the effectiveness of its suicide prevention media outreach campaign in raising such awareness, but has not established targets for the majority of these metrics because officials reported that there are no meaningful, industry-wide targets for them. We disagree with VHA's assertion that other targets would not be meaningful; VHA collects data on its metrics that it can use to develop reasonable and meaningful targets for future performance. In the absence of established targets, VHA cannot evaluate the effectiveness of the campaign, and make informed decisions about which activities should be continued to support VA's overall goal of reducing veteran suicides.

RECOMMENDATIONS FOR EXECUTIVE ACTION

We are making the following two recommendations to VA:

1. The Under Secretary for Health should establish an approach for overseeing its suicide prevention media outreach efforts that includes clear delineation of roles and responsibilities for those in leadership and contract oversight roles, including during periods of staff turnover or program changes (Recommendation 1).
2. The Under Secretary for Health should require officials within the Office of Suicide Prevention and Mental Health to establish targets for the metrics the office uses to evaluate the effectiveness of its suicide prevention media outreach campaign (Recommendation 2).

AGENCY COMMENTS AND OUR EVALUATION

We provided a draft of this chapter to VA for review and comment. In its written comments, summarized below and reprinted in Appendix I, VA concurred with our recommendations. VA described ongoing and planned actions and provided a timeline for addressing our recommendations. VA also provided technical comments, which we incorporated as appropriate.

In response to our first recommendation, to establish an oversight approach that includes delineation of roles and responsibilities, VA acknowledged that organizational transitions and realignments within OMHSP contributed to unclear roles and responsibilities in 2017 and 2018. VA said that OMHSP has made organizational improvements, including hiring a permanent Director for Suicide Prevention and establishing a new organizational structure. In its comments, VA requested closure of the first recommendation based on these actions. However, to fully implement this recommendation, VA will need to provide evidence that it has established an oversight approach for the suicide prevention media outreach campaign. This would include providing information about the roles and responsibilities, as well as reporting requirements, for contract and leadership officials involved in the suicide prevention media outreach campaign under the new organizational structure and the new contract. VA will also need to demonstrate that it has a plan in place to ensure continued oversight of the suicide prevention media campaign in the event of staff turnover or program changes. In response to our second recommendation, to establish targets against which to evaluate suicide prevention metrics, VA said it has plans to work with communications experts to develop metrics, targets, and an evaluation strategy to improve its evaluation of its suicide prevention program efforts, including outreach. VA expects to complete these actions by April 2019.

As agreed with your office, unless you publicly announce the contents of this chapter earlier, we plan no further distribution until 30 days from the report date. At that time, we will send copies to the appropriate congressional committees and the Secretary of Veterans Affairs.

Sincerely yours,

Debra A. Draper
Director, Health Care

APPENDIX I: COMMENTS FROM THE DEPARTMENT OF VETERANS AFFAIRS

THE SECRETARY OF VETERANS AFFAIRS
WASHINGTON

October 31, 2018

Ms. Debra A. Draper
Director
Health Care
U.S. Government Accountability Office
441 G Street, NW
Washington, DC 20548

Dear Ms. Draper:

The Department of Veterans Affairs (VA) has reviewed the Government Accountability Office (GAO) draft report: ***"VA HEALTH CARE: Improvements Needed in Suicide Prevention Media Outreach Oversight and Evaluation"*** (GAO-19-66).

The enclosure contains technical comments and sets forth the actions to be taken to address the draft report recommendations.

VA appreciates the opportunity to comment on your draft report.

Sincerely,

Robert L. Wilkie

Department of Veterans Affairs (VA) Comments to
Government Accountability Office (GAO) Draft Report
"VA HEALTH CARE: Improvements Needed in Suicide Prevention Media Outreach Campaign Oversight and Evaluation"
(GAO-19-66)

GAO Recommendation 1: The Under Secretary for Health should establish an approach for overseeing its suicide prevention media outreach efforts that includes delineation of roles and responsibilities for those in leadership and contract oversight roles, including during periods of staff turnover or program changes.

VA Comment: Concur. Suicide prevention is the Department of Veterans Affairs' (VA) highest priority. Every death by suicide is a tragedy, and we will not relent in our efforts to connect Veterans in need with life-saving support. VA's goal is to reduce suicide among Veterans. We can save lives.

VA's published National Strategy for Preventing Veteran Suicide provides the framework for identifying priorities, organizing efforts, and contributing to a national focus on Veteran suicide prevention over the next decade. The strategy aligns with the 2012 National Strategy for Suicide Prevention, consists of 4 strategic directions, 14 goals, 43 objectives, leverages the public health approach to suicide prevention, and focuses on the importance of collaboration and urgency.

The four strategic directions are:

1. Healthy and Empowered Veterans, Families, and Communities
   Work with community partners and policymakers to promote resources for Veterans and to promote mental health awareness and treatment.

2. Clinical and Community Preventive Services
   Share resources, training opportunities, interventions, and lethal means safety resources with providers outside VA and with clergy, first responders, law enforcement officials, and community partners.

3. Treatment, Recovery, and Support Services
   Work with local emergency departments and hospitals to promote Veteran suicide prevention resources and to ensure continuity of care for all Veterans admitted to an inpatient mental health unit.

4. Surveillance, Research, and Evaluation
   Share the VA National Suicide Data Report and National Strategy for Preventing Veteran Suicide with community partners.

VA has a comprehensive approach to suicide prevention. Here are just a few of our substantial efforts:

1. Expanding the Veterans Crisis Line that connects Veterans in crisis and their families and friends with qualified, caring VA responders through a confidential toll-free hotline, online chat, or text. Veterans and their loved ones can call **1-800-273-8255 and Press 1**, chat online, or send a text message to 838255 to receive confidential support 24 hours a day, 7 days a week, 365 days a year. More information is available at https://www.veteranscrisisline.net/.

2. Creating new cross-sector partnerships across various disciplines: faith communities, employers, schools, and health care organizations to name a few. Together we can reach more people.

3. Implementing the Joint Action Plan for Supporting Veterans During Their Transition From Uniformed Service to Civilian Life

4. Launching S.A.V.E. online suicide prevention training that educates yourself or your employees about how to recognize suicide risk factors and warning signs.

5. Implementing the Mayor's Challenge, which equips communities to build coalitions to prevent Veteran suicide. This partnership between VA and the Department of Health and Human Service Substance Abuse and Mental Health Services Administration (SAMHSA) helps local leaders in city governments work together to prevent suicide among Veterans. We have 27 Mayors now and we want more.

6. #BeThere prevention initiative teaches members of the community how simple acts can help save a Veteran in crisis. More information is available at https://www.veteranscrisisline.net/BeThere.aspx.

7. Make the Connection campaign is an online resource that connects Veterans, their family members and friends, and other supporters with information and solutions to issues affecting their lives. More information is available at https://maketheconnection.net/.

8. Coaching into Care (1-888-823-7458) is a national telephone service of VA. Coaching into Care aims to educate, support, and empower family members and friends who are seeking care or services for a Veteran. More information is available at https://www.mirecc.va.gov/coaching/.

9. Recovery Engagement and Coordination for Health – Veterans Enhanced Treatment Program (REACH VET) is an innovative program that applies principles of predictive medicine to prevent suicide.

10. About Face videos feature the real stories of Veterans who have experienced post-traumatic stress disorder with additional perspectives from their family members and VA clinicians. https://www.ptsd.va.gov/apps/AboutFace/.

11. How to Talk to a Child About a Suicide Attempt in Your Family: If there has been a recent suicide attempt in your family, this may be one of the toughest experiences you and your children may ever face. It is important to take care of yourself, so that you are better able to care for your child.

12. Paid media outreach such as advertisements on digital and social media.

VA's suicide prevention efforts are successful:

- Over 16,000 American citizens have downloaded VA's S.A.V.E. training to prevent suicides. Annual S.A.V.E. training is mandatory for VA employees, and in September 2018 alone over 52,000 VA employees completed it.

- The number of Veterans receiving mental health care in VA doubled over the past 10 years, now we are helping over 1.7 million Veterans with their mental health concerns.

- VA repeatedly meets our goals for being in the top 10 percent Nielsen ranking for our suicide prevention public service announcements.

- The Veterans Crisis Line serves about 2000 callers a day. Over the past 10 years, the Veterans Crisis Line has answered over 3 million calls, more than 363,000 online chats, and more than 83,000 text messages.

- Last year, VA's suicide prevention coordinators did 18,836 community outreach events and reached approximately 1,932,902 people.

- Over 102,000 people visited our #BeThere campaign page last year.

- Twenty-seven mayors are taking the challenge to reduce Veteran suicide in their cities. VA wants every city to take action to prevent suicide.

- During Suicide Prevention Month (September 2018) VA saw a lot of success with #BeThere messaging:

    - 50+ million #BeThere Twitter Chat impressions

- 18 million+ social media reach (over past 7 days)
- 2.6 million Thunderclap social media reach
- 1,800+ registrants for Action Alliance's Messaging Webinar
- 100+ private and public sector partners

In 2018, VA partnered with Johnson & Johnson on a broadly promoted public service announcement featuring Tom Hanks speaking that GAO did not include in the draft report. YouTube alone had over 30,000 views. VA showcased it as part of the #BeThere campaign. This outreach effort was supported through a non-monetary Memorandum of Agreement with Johnson & Johnson, at no cost to the Veterans Health Administration (VHA).

Regarding Paid Media spending, VHA estimates that the total amount spent in fiscal year (FY) 2018 will be about $1.5M. This will include money spent in September 2018 for Suicide Prevention Month paid media. VHA will not have final invoices for an exact total until sometime after October 2018. As indicated above, paid media is only one component of VHA's comprehensive suicide prevention effort, and it is a small portion of VHA's annual expenditures for suicide prevention.

VHA acknowledges that organizational transitions and realignments within Office of Mental Health and Suicide Prevention (OMHSP) contributed to unclear roles and responsibilities from mid-2017 to mid-2018. OMHSP has made significant organizational structure improvements to clearly delineate roles and responsibilities for those in leadership and contract oversight roles since that time. Organizational improvements within the Executive Leadership team and the Suicide Prevention team also ensure continuity during periods of staff turnover and program changes. OMHSP has hired a permanent Director for Suicide Prevention, and established and received approval for a permanent organizational structure which creates a clear chain of command within OMHSP and to VHA. With this new robust organizational structure in place, the Director for Suicide Prevention oversees communications and outreach activities in a more organized and deliberate manner. Similarly, contractual tasks related to these outreach activities fall within the Deputy Director for Partnerships' portfolio.

VHA has completed work on this recommendation and requests GAO close this recommendation as implemented. In support of our closure request, VHA has submitted the final, signed OMHSP organizational chart to GAO. Completion Date: July 2018

Recommendation 2: The Under Secretary for Health should require officials within the Office of Suicide Prevention and Mental Health to establish targets for the metrics the office uses to evaluate the effectiveness of its suicide prevention media outreach campaign.

VA Comment: Concur. GAO recognized that OMHSP has a robust monitoring process in place to track both reach and engagement of our suicide prevention outreach campaigns. Beyond quantitative data, OMHSP also tracks qualitative measures of success such as establishing partnerships with prominent organizations or securing promotion of our resources from high-profile public figures.

VHA has looked at broad indicators of impact for its suicide prevention outreach efforts for some time. VHA's current Agency Priority Goal is to provide core recommended interventions to Veterans targeted through its predictive risk modeling algorithms and to reduce Veteran suicide through a "Mayor's Challenge" partnership program. The growth in demand for services at the Veterans Crisis Line (VCL) has grown year over year and has been supported through ongoing outreach. In particular over FY 2018, the demand for chat and text services at VCL increased by over 25 percent and nearly 30 percent, respectively. Local outreach activities have also been part of national strategy including annual Community Mental Health Summits at VHA facilities. In 2018 there were 149 Summits with over 13,500 participants, and 83 percent of participants reported gaining a better understanding of suicide prevention resources and services through VHA and in their community.

VHA accepts GAO's recommendation to do more. OMHSP has begun to leverage VA expertise in health communication and evaluation to determine additional measures of effectiveness. These measures will be benchmarked against similar national program metrics. This effort is part of a larger initiative that is underway to determine program measures of effectiveness for the entire suicide prevention program. After receiving results from communications experts, OMHSP will finalize metrics, targets and the subsequent evaluation strategy. Target Completion Date: April 2019.

In: Improvements Needed in the VA … ISBN: 978-1-53615-971-4
Editor: Charles Copeland

Chapter 4

INDEPENDENT VERIFICATION AND VALIDATION OF PATIENT SELF-SCHEDULING SYSTEMS WAS CONSISTENT WITH THE FASTER CARE FOR VETERANS ACT OF 2016*

United States Government Accountability Office

June 13, 2018
Congressional Committees

The Faster Care for Veterans Act of 2016 called for the Department of Veterans Affairs (VA) to conduct a pilot program under which veterans can use an Internet website or mobile application to schedule and confirm appointments at the department's medical facilities.[1] The act also called for the department to hire a non-governmental, not-for-profit entity with expertise in health information technology to perform independent verification and validation (IV&V) of the patient self-scheduling system

* This is an edited, reformatted and augmented version of United States Government Accountability Office; Report to Congressional Requesters, Publication No. GAO-18-442R, dated June 2018.

[1] Pub. L. No. 114-286, §§ 2-3, 130 Stat. 1459-1461 (2016).

used in the pilot program, and any other patient self-scheduling system used by the department.[2] The IV&V was to determine whether the system or systems included seven minimum capabilities that are specified in the act to support the scheduling of medical appointments. VA subsequently contracted with the MITRE Corporation in April 2017 to conduct the IV&V.

The Faster Care for Veterans Act included a provision calling for us to evaluate the IV&V of VA's patient self-scheduling systems. Our specific objective was to determine if the IV&V included an evaluation of whether the systems provided the seven minimum capabilities specified in the act and was performed consistent with practices included in the Institute of Electrical and Electronics Engineers' (IEEE) Standard for System and Software Verification and Validation.[3]

To address the objective, we obtained and reviewed documentation, including VA's IV&V contract and performance work statement with MITRE, as well as the contractor's plans and final IV&V report. Specifically, we reviewed the findings in the final IV&V report with respect to VA's two patient self-scheduling systems—the On-line Patient Self Scheduling (OPSS) system and the Veteran Appointment Request (VAR) system—and their inclusion of the seven minimum capabilities called for in the act. We did not independently determine whether OPSS and VAR included the minimum capabilities. However, we evaluated the MITRE report to see if it addressed the use of applicable practices identified in the IEEE standard, including practices for ensuring independence, as well as those related to software, system, and hardware validation and verification.

We supplemented our analysis with interviews of relevant VA and MITRE officials to gain an understanding of the work that was performed

[2] The purpose of IV&V is to provide an independent review of system processes and products to ensure that quality standards are being met. The use of IV&V is a recognized best practice for system development and acquisition programs and involves an independent organization conducting unbiased reviews of processes, products, and results to verify and validate that they meet stated requirements and standards.

[3] Institute of Electrical and Electronics Engineers, *IEEE Standard for System and Software Verification and Validation,* IEEE Std. 1012-2012 (New York, N.Y., May 25, 2012). Adapted and reprinted with permission from IEEE. Copyright IEEE 2012. All rights reserved.

to complete the IV&V. These included officials in VA's Office of Quality, Privacy, and Risk within the Office of Information and Technology, as well as MITRE's project leader and other IV&V report authors. Additionally, we viewed demonstrations of the OPSS and VAR systems.[4]

We conducted this performance audit from December 2017 to June 2018 in accordance with generally accepted government auditing standards. Those standards require that we plan and perform the audit to obtain sufficient, appropriate evidence to provide a reasonable basis for our findings and conclusions based on our audit objectives. We believe that the evidence obtained provides a reasonable basis for our findings and conclusions based on our audit objectives.

BACKGROUND

VA operates the largest health care delivery system in the United States, providing health care to 7 million veterans and their families at more than 1,500 medical facilities. At these facilities, the department provides outpatient care through primary and specialty care clinics. According to VA's fiscal year 2019 congressional budget submission, it expects nearly 118 million outpatient visits from veterans for primary and specialty care.

However, we and others have previously expressed concerns about VA's ability to effectively provide and oversee timely access to health care. For example, we have reported on persistent issues with scheduling patients' medical appointments at the department.[5] Based on patient

---

[4] VAR was renamed the VA Online Scheduling system in December 2017, but at the time of the IV&V was named VAR.

[5] See, for example, GAO, *VA Health Care: Reliability of Reported Outpatient Medical Appointment Wait Times and Scheduling Oversight Need Improvement*, GAO-13-130 (Washington, D.C.: Dec. 21, 2012); *VA Health Care: Management and Oversight of Consult Process Need Improvement to Help Ensure Veterans Receive Timely Outpatient Specialty Care,* GAO-14-808 (Washington, D.C.: Sept. 30, 2014); and *VA Mental Health: Clearer Guidance on Access Policies and Wait-Time Data Needed,* GAO-16-24 (Washington, D.C.: Oct. 28, 2015). See also Department of Veterans Affairs, Office of Inspector General, *Healthcare Inspection: Gastroenterology Consult Delays, William Jennings Bryan Dorn VA Medical Center, Columbia, South Carolina,* Report No. 12-04631-313 (Washington, D.C.: Sept. 6, 2013); and Department of Veterans Affairs, Office of Inspector General, *Veterans Health Administration, Review of Alleged Patient Deaths, Patient Wait Times, and*

scheduling problems and other serious and longstanding concerns about the department's management and oversight of its health care system, we added VA health care to GAO's High Risk List in 2015.[6]

The Faster Care for Veterans Act specified seven minimum capabilities that are to be provided by VA's systems used to support patient self-scheduling of medical appointments. These include the capabilities to schedule, modify, and cancel appointments; support both in-person and telehealth appointments;[7] view appointment availability in real time; and integrate with the department's health information system—the Veterans Health Information Systems and Technology Architecture (VistA). Table 1 lists the seven minimum capabilities called for in the act.

Table 1. List of Capabilities that the Faster Care for Veterans Act of 2016 Required the Department of Veterans Affairs to Include in Patient Self-Scheduling Systems

Schedule, modify, and cancel appointments for primary care, specialty care, and mental health.
Support appointments for the provision of health care regardless of whether such care is provided in person or through telehealth services.
View appointment availability in real time.
Make available, in real time, appointments that were previously filled, but later canceled, by other patients.
Provide prompts or reminders to veterans to schedule follow-up appointments.
Be available for use 24 hours per day, 7 days per week.
Integrate with the Veterans Health Information Systems and Technology Architecture (VistA), or such successor information technology system.

Source: Faster Care for Veterans Act of 2016. | GAO-18-442R.

In April 2017, VA initiated the pilot patient self-scheduling program called for in the Faster Care for Veterans Act of 2016. The pilot program included the acquisition of OPSS, which the department implemented beginning in December 2017 to allow veterans to use an Internet website or

Scheduling Practices at the Phoenix VA Health Care System, Report No. 14-02603-267 (Washington, D.C.: Aug. 26, 2014).

[6] GAO, *High Risk Series: An Update*, GAO-15-290, (Washington, D.C.: Feb. 11, 2015).

[7] Telehealth includes telemedicine, which is the use of medical information exchanged from one site to another via electronic communications (such as video or e-mail) to improve a patient's clinical health status through, for example, provision of health care services or clinical monitoring.

mobile application to schedule appointments at three VA medical centers. In addition, prior to the enactment of the Faster Care for Veterans Act, the department had developed VAR as a system that also was to be used to support appointment self-scheduling. The department began national deployment of VAR in January 2017 and, as of December 2017, had deployed the system at 111 VA medical centers. The act did not specify that existing systems, such as VAR, were to be included in the pilot program, but it did state that such systems were required to meet the seven minimum capabilities and were subject to the IV&V requirement of the act.

Also in April 2017, VA entered into a contract with MITRE to conduct the IV&V called for in the act. MITRE is a non-governmental, not-for-profit entity with expertise in health information technology that operates multiple federally funded research and development centers and conducts work with VA to address the challenges of providing seamless, timely delivery of benefits and services to veterans. MITRE completed its IV&V report on VAR and OPSS in February 2018.

Independent Verification and Validation of VA's Patient Self-Scheduling Systems Included an Evaluation of Capabilities Specified in the Faster Care for Veterans Act of 2016 and Was Performed Consistent with IEEE Practices

The IV&V that MITRE performed for OPSS and VAR included findings on whether the two systems met each of the seven minimum capabilities called for in the Faster Care for Veterans Act of 2016. The IV&V findings on the extent to which the systems provided the seven capabilities, including strengths and weaknesses as reported by MITRE, are identified in Table 2.

Table 2: MITRE Independent Validation and Verification Findings on the Department of Veterans Affairs' (VA) Patient Self-Scheduling Appointment Systems

Capability identified in the Faster Care for Veterans Act of 2016	Finding for the Veteran Appointment Request (VAR) System	Finding for the On-line Patient Self-Scheduling System (OPSS)
Schedule, modify, and cancel appointments for primary care, specialty care, and mental health.	The system provided capabilities to schedule and cancel appointments, but did not provide the capability to modify appointments.	The system provided these capabilities, but did not operate as expected for mental health appointments.
Support appointments for the provision of health care regardless of whether such care is provided in person or through telehealth services.	The system provided the capability for veterans to self-schedule in person appointments. Telehealth appointments requested by veterans were not directly scheduled by veterans.	The system did not provide an ability to directly schedule telehealth appointments.
View appointment availability in real time.	The system accurately provided this capability for the services that VA offers veterans to directly schedule appointments.	The system accurately but inconsistently provided this capability for the services that VA offers veterans to directly schedule appointments.
Make available, in real time, appointments that were previously filled but later canceled by other patients.	Previously scheduled appointments, when canceled, were accurately presented as available in the user interface in real time.	Previously scheduled appointments, when canceled, were accurately presented as available in the user interface in real time.
Provide prompts or reminders to veteran to schedule follow-up appointments.	The system provided this capability in the form of "Notifications" in the user interface. The system integrated with the VA Recall Reminder system to provide veterans with such notifications.	The system did not operate as expected when providing veterans with prompts or reminders to schedule follow up appointments.
Be available for use 24 hours per day, 7 days per week	There was minimal information provided or found as evidence (e.g., operational up-time/down-time, failure statistics, and recovery ability) of the system's ability to reliably operate 24x7 under expected operational conditions, such as expected and peak loads; upgrades; and faults with the system, networks, and integrated systems.	There was minimal information provided or found as evidence (e.g., operational up-time/down-time, failure statistics, and recovery ability) of the system's ability to reliably operate 24x7 under expected operational conditions, such as expected and peak loads; upgrades; and faults with the system, networks, and integrated systems.

Capability identified in the Faster Care for Veterans Act of 2016	**Finding for the Veteran Appointment Request (VAR) System**	**Finding for the On-line Patient Self-Scheduling System (OPSS)**
Integrate with the Veterans Health Information Systems and Technology Architecture (VistA), or such successor information technology system.	The system's integration with VistA resulted in accurate real time data being presented to users. VAR's architecture was observed to be adaptable for integrating with potential future successor systems.	The system's integration with VistA resulted in some data being accurately presented to users. However, OPSS does not receive complete scheduling and reminder data from VistA.

Source: MITRE IV&V report on VA Patient Self-Scheduling Appointment Systems for the Faster Care for Veterans Act of 2016. | GAO-18-442R.

Independent Verification and Validation was Consistent with the IEEE Standard

In addition to addressing whether OPSS and VAR included the minimum requirements called for in the Faster Care for Veterans Act, the IV&V conducted by MITRE was consistent with the IEEE standard for performing such evaluations. Specifically, this standard recommends that an IV&V be performed by personnel who are not involved in the development of the system under evaluation. Additionally, the standard specifies that managerial and financial responsibility for the IV&V be placed in an organization separate from the system development and program management organizations.

We determined that VA and MITRE took appropriate steps to ensure independence of the contractor's staff who conducted the IV&V. Specifically, VA assigned the task order for the IV&V to an office in the department that was separate from the organization that managed other work MITRE was performing. Additionally, the MITRE staff that worked on the IV&V were fully dedicated to the effort and did not work on other task orders that the organization held with VA. Further, the MITRE IV&V team was not involved in supporting the development of VAR or the acquisition of OPSS. Lastly, MITRE asserted in its IV&V report for the two systems, that all assessment criteria for the IV&V were developed and assessed independent of VA and of the product teams for the systems evaluated.

The IV&V also was consistent with the IEEE standard for conducting verification and validation activities. This standard calls for the IV&V to, among other things, include activities that are grouped into three verification and validation areas: system verification and validation, software verification and validation, and hardware verification and validation. The IV&V that MITRE performed for OPSS and VAR addressed each of the specific activities in the three areas outlined in the standard, as discussed in detail below.

With regard to system verification and validation, the IEEE standard identifies seven activities that are to be performed, as listed in Table 3.

The IV&V for OPSS and VAR indicates that MITRE addressed all seven system verification and validation activities described in the IEEE standard. For example, MITRE's report indicated that the IV&V addressed the requirements analysis verification and validation activity by analyzing the seven minimum requirements for self-scheduling appointment systems specified in the Faster Care for Veterans Act. In addition, MITRE's report provided evidence that the IV&V assessed whether stakeholder requirements were traceable to the originating stakeholders. MITRE's report also indicated that the IV&V addressed the maintenance verification and validation activity by evaluating whether the VAR and OPSS support mechanisms included long-term sustainment actions, such as monitoring system performance and providing administrative support.

With respect to software verification and validation, the IEEE standard identifies 10 activities that are to be performed. These activities are listed in Table 4.

The IV&V for OPSS and VAR indicates that MITRE addressed all 10 software verification and validation activities identified in the IEEE standard. For instance, MITRE's report indicated that it addressed the software requirements verification and validation activity by assessing OPSS's and VAR's capabilities against those called for in the Faster Care for Veterans Act. MITRE's report also provided evidence that the IV&V evaluated test cases and design scenarios for the systems to address this activity. Further, MITRE's report indicated that the IV&V addressed the software design verification and validation activity by conducting design observation scenarios to provide insight into the level of quality and completeness of functionality when the systems were in a production environment using scheduling data. The software acceptance test activity was addressed by conducting analyses of test cases, including user acceptance testing, that compared test cases to the requirements of OPSS and VAR.

Table 3. Institute of Electrical and Electronics Engineers Standard for System Verification and Validation (V&V) Activities

Verification and validation standard activities
Requirements analysis V&V includes an assessment of whether the system requirements specify all required characteristics for the system.
Stakeholder requirements definition V&V includes an assessment of whether the stakeholder requirements are traceable to the originating stakeholders.
Architectural design V&V assures that the architecture satisfies the system requirements.
Implementation V&V verifies that the implementation activities performed produces a system that conforms to the system requirements.
Integration V&V assures that the system integration strategy is consistent with the system architecture.
Transition V&V assesses that the system is installed in its operational location in accordance with the transition plan.
Maintenance V&V is to assess that the maintenance strategy is comprehensive and explicitly documented.

Source: Institute of Electrical and Electronics Engineers | GAO-18-442R.

Note: IEEE Standard for System and Software Verification and Validation, IEEE Std. 1012-2012 (New York, N.Y., May 25, 2012). Adapted and reprinted with permission from IEEE.

With regard to hardware verification and validation, the IEEE standard specifies 10 activities that are intended to verify that hardware components satisfy the hardware specifications. These 10 hardware verification and validation activities are listed in Table 5.

The IV&V for OPSS and VAR indicates that MITRE addressed all 10 of the hardware verification and validation activities described in the IEEE standard, including the hardware integration test verification and validation activity. This activity calls for a determination of whether hardware conforms to requirements during the integration process.

Table 4. Institute of Electrical and Electronics Engineers Standard for Software Verification and Validation (V&V)

Verification and validation standard activities
Software concept V&V verifies the allocation of system requirements, validate the selected solution, and assure that no false assumptions have been incorporated in the solution.
Software requirements V&V assures the correctness, completeness, accuracy, testability, and consistency of the system software requirements.
Software design V&V demonstrates that the design is a correct, accurate, and complete transformation of the software requirements and that no unintended features are introduced.
Software construction V&V verifies and validates that the system design that is transformed into code is correct, accurate, and complete.
Software integration test V&V assures that the software requirements and system requirements allocated to software are validated as each software component is incrementally integrated.
Software qualification test V&V assures that the integrated software product satisfies its requirements.
Software acceptance test V&V assures that the software satisfies its acceptance criteria and to enable the customer to determine whether or not to accept the integrated software product.
Software installation and checkout V&V verifies and validates the correctness of the software installation in the target environment.
Software operation V&V assesses the proposed system changes and their impact on the software, and evaluate the operating procedures for correctness and usability.
Software maintenance V&V assesses the proposed software system changes and their impact on the software.

Source: Institute of Electrical and Electronics Engineers | GAO-18-442R.

Note: IEEE Standard for System and Software Verification and Validation, IEEE Std. 1012-2012 (New York, N.Y., May 25, 2012). Adapted and reprinted with permission from IEEE. Copyright IEEE 2012. All rights reserved.

MITRE's report indicated that the IV&V addressed this activity by evaluating whether the two systems integrated with VistA and other data sources needed for scheduling appointments and clinical data exchange. In addition, MITRE's report provided evidence that the IV&V addressed the hardware transition verification and validation activity by determining whether the scheduling systems supported mechanisms to ensure proper initial operation and sustainment. Hardware design verification and validation was also addressed in the IV&V by checking the level of quality and completeness of functionality when the scheduling systems were used with live patient scheduling data on the VA network.

Table 5. Institute of Electrical and Electronics Engineers Standard for Hardware Verification and Validation (V&V)

Verification and validation standard activities
Hardware concept V&V verifies that all system requirements allocated to the hardware components are addressed and validates that the selected hardware concepts satisfy the system needs.
Hardware requirements V&V verifies that the hardware requirements correctly, completely, and accurately satisfy the system requirements allocated to the hardware element and validates that the hardware requirements, in total, satisfy the system needs.
Hardware design V&V verifies that all hardware design components satisfy the hardware requirements specification of the hardware element.
Hardware fabrication V&V verifies that the final fabrication elements comply with the hardware design and to validate that each fabricated hardware component satisfies the overall system performance, safety, and reliability requirements.
Hardware integration test V&V verifies that hardware parts conform to the hardware element requirements during the integration process and validates that the hardware element satisfies the system requirements.
Hardware qualification test V&V verifies that the hardware element as tested satisfies the hardware requirements and validates that the hardware element satisfies system requirements.
Hardware acceptance test V&V verifies that the hardware element meets the acceptance criteria and requirements and validates that the system requirements allocated to this particular hardware element are satisfied.
Hardware transition V&V verifies and validates the correctness of the hardware installation in the operational environment.
Hardware operation V&V assesses proposed system changes and their impact on the hardware and evaluate operating procedures for correctness and usability.
Hardware maintenance V&V assesses proposed hardware changes and their impact on the system.

Source: Institute of Electrical and Electronics Engineers | GAO-18-442R.

Note: IEEE Standard for System and Software Verification and Validation, IEEE Std. 1012-2012 (New York, N.Y., May 25, 2012). Adapted and reprinted with permission from IEEE. Copyright IEEE 2012. All rights reserved.

AGENCY COMMENTS AND OUR EVALUATION

VA provided written comments on a draft of this chapter, which are reprinted in the enclosure. In its comments, the department concurred with our assessment that MITRE's IV&V was performed consistent with the IEEE standards for software, system, and hardware verification and validation.

The department also agreed with our determination that the IV&V had reviewed whether VAR and OPSS included the seven minimum capabilities specified in the Faster Care for Veterans Act.

We are sending copies of this chapter to the Committees on Veterans' Affairs of the Senate and the House of Representatives and the Committees on Appropriations, Subcommittees on Military Construction, Veterans Affairs, and Related Agencies, of the Senate and the House of Representatives; and to the Acting Secretary of Veterans Affairs.

David A. Powner
Director, Information Technology Management Issues

ENCLOSURE

DEPARTMENT OF VETERANS AFFAIRS
WASHINGTON DC 20420

May 29, 2018

David A. Powner
Director
Information Technology Management Issues
U.S. Government Accountability Office
441 G Street, NW
Washington, DC 20548

Dear Mr. Powner:

The Department of Veterans Affairs (VA) has reviewed the Government Accountability Office's (GAO) draft report, ***"VA HEALTH CARE: Independent Verification and Validation of Patient Self-Scheduling Systems Was Consistent with the Faster Care for Veterans Act of 2016"*** (GAO-18-442R).

The enclosure provides our general comment. VA appreciates the opportunity to comment on your draft report.

Sincerely,

Peter M. O'Rourke
Chief of Staff

Department of Veterans Affairs (VA) Comments to
Government Accountability Office (GAO) Draft Report
"VA HEALTH CARE: Independent Verification and Validation of Patient Self-Scheduling Systems Was Consistent with the Faster Care for Veterans Act of 2016"
(GAO-18-442R)

General Comment:

The Government Accountability Office's (GAO) Draft Report titled ***"VA HEALTH CARE: Independent Verification and Validation of Patient Self-Scheduling Systems Was Consistent with the Faster Care for Veterans Act of 2016"*** (GAO-18-442R) listed two specific GAO objectives. The first was that the MITRE independent verification and validation (IV&V) was performed consistent with practices included in the Institute of Electrical and Electronics Engineers' (IEEE) standards for System, Software, and Hardware verification and validation (V&V). The Veterans Health Administration (VHA) concurs that MITRE's IV&V met the IEEE standards for System, Software, and Hardware V&V.

The second objective was to determine if the MITRE IV&V included an evaluation of whether the Veteran Appointment Request (VAR) (now known as VA Online Scheduling) and the Online Patient Self-Scheduling (OPSS) systems provided the seven minimum capabilities specified in the Act. VHA agrees that MITRE reviewed the seven minimum capabilities for VAR and OPSS and judged their compliance based on IV&V standards.

Using these standards, MITRE reported telehealth capability was not observed with OPSS. While VA appreciates MITRE had to use the IV&V standards to judge the telehealth standard accordingly, the capability for OPSS to make telehealth appointments does exist. At the time of the MITRE assessment, the OPSS systems pilot was less than 60 days old and the OPSS software was deployed to limited clinics at 3 pilot sites. Although available, the sites had not yet set-up the clinic profiles to demonstrate telehealth appointing at that time. VA wishes to assure the public that the seven capabilities required by the Act do in fact exist.

List of Committees

The Honorable Johnny Isakson
Chairman

The Honorable Jon Tester
Ranking Member
Committee on Veterans' Affairs
United States Senate

The Honorable John Boozman
Chairman

The Honorable Brian Schatz
Ranking Member
Subcommittee on Military Construction, Veterans Affairs, and Related Agencies Committee on Appropriations
United States Senate

The Honorable Phil Roe
Chairman

The Honorable Tim Walz
Ranking Member
Committee on Veterans' Affairs
House of Representatives

The Honorable John Carter
Chairman

The Honorable Debbie Wasserman Schultz
Ranking Member
Subcommittee on Military Construction, Veterans Affairs, and Related Agencies Committee on Appropriations
House of Representatives

In: Improvements Needed in the VA … ISBN: 978-1-53615-971-4
Editor: Charles Copeland

Chapter 5

IMPROVED OVERSIGHT NEEDED FOR REUSABLE MEDICAL EQUIPMENT*

United States Government Accountability Office

ABBREVIATIONS

RME	reusable medical equipment
SPS	Sterile Processing Service
VA	Department of Veterans Affairs
VAMC	VA medical center
VHA	Veterans Health Administration
VISN	Veterans Integrated Service Network

WHY GAO DID THIS STUDY

VHA operates one of the largest health care delivery systems in the nation, serving over 9 million enrolled veterans. In providing health care

* This is an edited, reformatted and augmented version of United States Government Accountability Office; Report to Congressional Requesters, Publication No. GAO-18-474, dated August 2018.

services to veterans, VAMCs use RME which must be reprocessed—that is, cleaned, disinfected, or sterilized— between uses. Improper reprocessing of RME can negatively affect patient care. To help ensure the safety of veterans, VHA policy establishes requirements VAMCs must follow when reprocessing RME and requires a number of related oversight efforts.

GAO was asked to review VHA's reprocessing of RME. This chapter examines (1) VHA's oversight of VAMCs' adherence to RME policies and (2) challenges VAMCs face in operating their Sterile Processing Services programs, and any efforts by VHA to address these challenges. GAO reviewed relevant VHA documents including RME policies and VISN inspection results for fiscal year 2017. GAO interviewed officials from VHA, all 18 VISNs, and four VAMCs, selected based on geographic variation, VAMC complexity, and data on operating room delays. GAO examined VHA's oversight in the context of federal internal control standards on communication, monitoring, and information.

What GAO Recommends

GAO is making three recommendations to VHA, including that it ensure all RME inspections are being conducted and complete results reported, and that it examine Sterile Processing Services workforce needs and make adjustments, as appropriate. VA concurred with these recommendations.

What GAO Found

GAO found that the Department of Veterans Affairs' (VA) Veterans Health Administration (VHA) does not have reasonable assurance that VA Medical Centers (VAMC) are following policies related to reprocessing reusable medical equipment (RME). Reprocessing involves cleaning, sterilizing, and storing surgical instruments and other RME, such as endoscopes. VHA has not ensured that all VAMCs' RME inspections have been conducted because it has incomplete information from the annual inspections by Veterans Integrated Service Networks (VISN), which oversee VAMCs. For fiscal year 2017, VHA did not have 39 of the 144 VISN reports from the VISNs' inspections of their VAMCs' Sterile Processing Services departments. VISNs were able to provide GAO with evidence that they had conducted 27 of the 39 missing inspections; top areas of non-adherence in these inspections were related to quality and training, among other things. Although VHA has ultimate oversight responsibility, a VHA official told GAO that VHA had not been aware it lacked complete inspection results because it has largely relied on the VISNs to ensure complete inspection result reporting. Without analyzing and sharing complete information from inspections, VHA does not have assurance that its VAMCs are following RME policies designed to ensure that veterans receive safe care.

GAO also found that VAMCs face challenges operating their Sterile Processing Services programs—notably, addressing workforce needs. Almost all of the officials from all 18 VISNs and selected VAMCs GAO interviewed reported Sterile Processing Services workforce challenges, such as lengthy hiring timeframes and limited pay and professional growth potential. According to officials, these challenges result in programs having difficulty maintaining sufficient staffing. VHA officials told GAO that the office is considering studying Sterile Processing Services staffing at VAMCs, although VHA does not have definitive plans to do so. VHA's Sterile Processing Services workforce challenges pose a potential risk to VAMCs' ability to ensure access to sterilized medical equipment, and VHA's failure to address this risk is inconsistent with standards for internal control in the federal government. Until VHA examines these workforce needs, VHA won't know whether or to what extent the reported challenges adversely affect VAMCs' ability to effectively operate their Sterile Processing Services programs and ensure access to safe care for veterans.

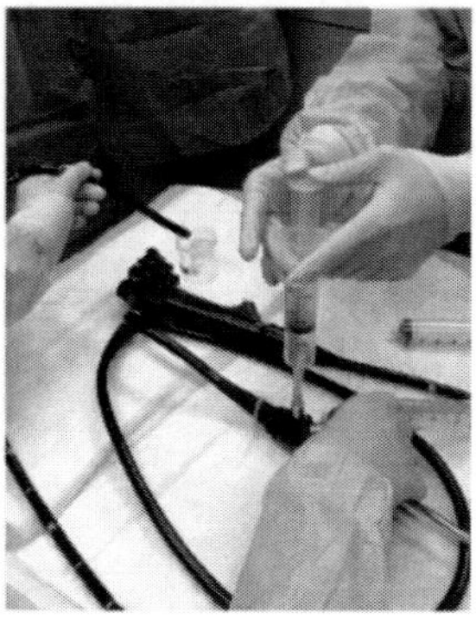

Source: Image of endoscope reprinted with permission from Ofstead & Associates, Inc. | GAO-18-474.

An endoscope is a kind of reusable medical equipment.

August 3, 2018

The Honorable Phil Roe
Chairman
Committee on Veterans' Affairs
House of Representatives

Dear Mr. Chairman:

The Department of Veterans Affairs' (VA) Veterans Health Administration (VHA) operates one of the largest health care delivery systems in the nation, serving over 9 million enrolled veterans. In providing health care services to veterans, VA medical centers (VAMC) use reusable medical equipment (RME), such as endoscopes and surgical instruments, which must be reprocessed—that is, cleaned, disinfected, or sterilized— between uses.[1] As medical instruments have become more complex, reprocessing has become more complicated and time consuming. For example, reprocessing an endoscope after a colonoscopy requires eight detailed cleaning steps and, on average, over 1 hour and 15 minutes of

[1] An endoscope is an instrument used for direct visual inspection of hollow organs or body cavities.

hands-on staff time.[2] Improper reprocessing of RME creates risks to patient safety—exposing patients to infection, for example—and can adversely affect timely access to care, such as when surgeries are delayed or canceled due to the lack of properly reprocessed medical equipment. The reprocessing of RME occurs at VAMCs within their Sterile Processing Services (SPS) programs.[3] To help ensure the safety of veterans who receive care at its facilities, VHA policy establishes requirements VAMCs must follow when reprocessing RME. Further, VHA policy requires inspections to be completed each year to determine the extent to which VAMCs are following these RME requirements and that incidents involving improperly reprocessed RME are reported. VHA has had ongoing challenges with RME reprocessing. For example, in 2009, two VAMCs notified about 10,000 veterans of their potential exposure to hepatitis B, hepatitis C, and HIV, because they received care using improperly reprocessed endoscopes.[4] In 2011 we found that VHA had not provided sufficient guidance to VAMC staff operating the SPS programs to ensure that staff were reprocessing RME correctly, which posed potential safety risks to veterans.[5] In 2016, the VHA Office of the Medical Inspector reviewed and corroborated allegations that the SPS department at a VAMC failed to provide surgeons with RME free of bioburden, debris, or both.[6] Further, in March 2018, the VA Office of Inspector General reported on problems at a VAMC that included RME- specific issues, such as delays

---

[2] See International Association of Healthcare Central Service Materiel Management Communique', *A Glimpse at the True Cost of Reprocessing Endoscopes: Results of a Pilot Project,* (Chicago, IL: January/February 2017).

[3] The VAMC SPS programs consist of the SPS department, which has primary responsibility for reprocessing RME, and other areas such as dental clinics, where certain reprocessing functions occur.

[4] See VA Office of Inspector General, *Healthcare Inspection: Use and Reprocessing of Flexible Fiberoptic Endoscopes at VA Medical Facilities*, (Washington, D.C.: June 16, 2009).

[5] See GAO, *VA Health Care: Weaknesses in Policies and Oversight Governing Medical Supplies and Equipment Pose Risks to Veterans' Safety*, GAO-11-391 (Washington, D.C.: May 3, 2011).

[6] Bioburden is a measure of microorganism contamination on an object. See Department of Veterans Affairs, *Department of Veterans Affairs Cincinnati Veterans Affairs Medical Center Cincinnati, Ohio, Veterans Integrated Service Network 10,* TRIM 2016-D-1082 (Washington, D.C.: May 8, 2016).

and cancellations of procedures due to unavailable instruments because of improper reprocessing.[7]

You asked us to review RME reprocessing within VHA. In this chapter, we examine:

1. VHA's oversight of VAMCs' adherence to RME policies and
2. challenges VAMCs face in operating their SPS programs, and any efforts by VHA to address these challenges.

To examine VHA's oversight, we assessed its efforts to oversee VHA's 18 Veterans Integrated Service Networks (VISN) and its efforts to directly ensure that VHA's 170 VAMCs are adhering to RME policies.[8] We reviewed VHA Directive 1116(2), which describes RME policy requirements and instructions for how inspections of VAMCs' adherence to these requirements should be conducted, and VHA's guide to issue briefs, which are reports that provide information on incidents involving improperly processed RME.[9] We reviewed summary data from VHA on inspections of VAMCs conducted by their respective VISNs in fiscal year 2017.[10] These summary data came from inspection reports submitted to VHA by the VISNs for which VHA had records as of February 2018. We also reviewed the full inspection reports that we obtained from the VISNs for inspections VISNs had conducted in fiscal year 2017, but for which

---

[7] See Department of Veterans Affairs, Office of Inspector General, Veterans Health Administration. *Critical Deficiencies at the Washington DC VA Medical Center.* Report #17-02644-130. (Washington, D.C.: March 7, 2018.)

[8] Each of the 18 VISNs is responsible for ensuring adherence to VHA's policies at the VAMCs within its region.

[9] See VHA Directive 1116(2), *Sterile Processing Services (SPS)* (Washington, D.C.: March 23, 2016). See Department of Veterans Affairs, Deputy Undersecretary for Health for Operations and Management (10N), *10N Guide to VHA Issue Briefs* (Washington, D.C.: June 26, 2017).

[10] VISNs and VAMCs are each required to conduct inspections to determine the extent of VAMCs' adherence to RME policy requirements annually. According to VHA officials, VHA also inspects each VAMC triennially. We focused our review on VISN inspection results because these inspections allowed us to determine the extent of adherence to RME-related requirements for all VAMCs for the most recent fiscal year at the time of our review, and because the inspections represent a level of oversight above VAMCs' own internal reviews. We reviewed inspection results for the SPS, dental, and gastroenterology areas in the VAMCs and did not include inspection results for satellite facilities such as community-based outpatient centers and health care centers.

VHA did not have records, which identified information about non-adherence to RME policy requirements.[11] Finally, we reviewed VHA's summary of issue briefs, including those related to the improper reprocessing of RME, for fiscal years 2015 through 2017.[12]

To assess the reliability of the inspection and issue brief data, we reviewed the data to identify missing information and discrepancies, and we interviewed VHA officials regarding the processes for collecting and verifying the data. Based on these efforts, we determined that VHA data on the number of VISN inspection reports for which they had records, VISN inspection reports, and VHA summary data from issue briefs were reliable for the purposes of our reporting objectives. In addition to our review of inspection and issue brief data, we interviewed VHA, VISN, and VAMC officials. Specifically, we interviewed VHA officials from the National Program Office for Sterile Processing, which is responsible for developing RME policies and overseeing VAMCs' adherence to these policies. We also interviewed officials from the 18 VISNs and four selected VAMCs to get their views on VHA's oversight.[13] We assessed VHA's oversight efforts in the context of federal standards for internal control for monitoring, information, and communication.[14]

---

[11] We also reviewed VHA's summary data for the other inspections conducted in 2017, but determined the summary data were not sufficiently reliable to report detailed information on the extent of VAMCs' non-adherence to RME policy requirements.

[12] We reviewed VISN inspection data for fiscal year 2017 because it was the most recent complete year of data available. We reviewed issue briefs for fiscal years 2015 through 2017 to ensure we had a sufficient sample.

[13] We selected the four VAMCs to achieve geographic and VAMC complexity variation and the highest and lowest performance regarding operating room lag time. VHA assigns each VAMC to one of five complexity groups based on patient population served, clinical services offered, education and research complexity, and administrative complexity. Operating room lag time data captures the time elapsed from one patient leaving and the next patient entering the operating room; lag time can be attributed to RME not being available, among other factors. The four VAMCs we selected were located in Chicago, IL; Erie, PA; Fort Meade, SD; and Little Rock, AR. Within the VAMCs, we spoke with officials from the SPS department, operating room, and gastroenterology and dental clinics. We were not able to speak with the Chief of SPS at the Chicago Jesse-Brown VAMC; as such, some of our reported results are for three VAMCs.

[14] See GAO, *Standards for Internal Control in the Federal Government,* GAO-14-704G (Washington, D.C.: September 2014). Internal control is a process effected by an entity's oversight body, management, and other personnel that provides reasonable assurance that the objectives of an entity will be achieved.

To examine challenges VAMCs face in operating their SPS programs, we reviewed VHA's RME policy and other documents to identify the requirements VAMCs must follow in operating their SPS programs, and we interviewed officials with direct knowledge of these efforts at all 18 VISNs and the four selected VAMCs. In addition, we asked operating room nurse managers from 20 selected VAMCs to identify in writing any RME-related challenges they faced as a result of the SPS department at their VAMC, such as delays in operating room procedures due to RME issues.[15] We discussed the challenges identified with officials from VHA's National Program Office for Sterile Processing and the Workforce Management and Consulting Office. We assessed VHA's efforts to address RME-related challenges in the context of federal standards for internal control for risk assessment.[16]

Finally, to provide a contextual understanding of RME issues across both objectives, we visited a VAMC with a large SPS program and interviewed officials outside of VHA with relevant knowledge. Specifically, we conducted an in-person site visit at the Seattle VAMC and spoke to officials involved in the SPS program, such as the SPS Chief and staff, VAMC leadership, and the Chief of Surgery and operating room Nurse Manager. Further, we spoke with officials from organizations with RME industry knowledge, such as the International Association of Healthcare Central Service Materiel Management and the Association for the Advancement of Medical Instrumentation—two professional associations that set RME reprocessing standards used by VHA and others, offer RME certification, and provide information and support regarding RME reprocessing to those working in the industry.[17] We also interviewed

---

[15] We selected the 20 VAMCs based on operating room lag time data. Of the 20 VAMCs, we selected 10 VAMCs with the lowest performance based on VA's operating room lag time data and 10 VAMCs with the highest performance based on these data. The 20 VAMCs we selected are located in West Los Angeles, CA; Beckley, WV; Martinez, CA; Chicago-Jesse Brown, IL; Fort Meade, SD; Portland, OR; St. Louis, MO; New Orleans, LA; Albuquerque, NM; Vieira, FL; Little Rock, AR; Billings, MT; Lake City, FL; St. Cloud, MN; Fargo, ND; Evansville, IN; Marion, IL; Erie, PA; Grand Junction, CO; and San Juan, PR. We did not receive responses from Billings, MT and San Juan, PR.

[16] See GAO-14-704G.

[17] RME certification is intended to ensure that RME professionals possess the essential knowledge and skills necessary for managing SPS tasks.

officials from the Joint Commission and the VA Office of Inspector General who periodically review VAMCs' SPS programs and contacted three Veterans Service Organizations to obtain their views on concerns related to RME reprocessing and suggestions for addressing those concerns.[18]

We conducted this performance audit from April 2017 to June 2018 in accordance with generally accepted government auditing standards. Those standards require that we plan and perform the audit to obtain sufficient, appropriate evidence to provide a reasonable basis for our findings and conclusions based on our audit objectives. We believe that the evidence obtained provides a reasonable basis for our findings and conclusions based on our audit objectives.

BACKGROUND

In providing health care services to veterans, clinicians at VAMCs use RME, such as endoscopes and surgical instruments, which must be reprocessed between uses. Reprocessing covers a wide range of instruments and has become increasingly complex. VHA has developed policies that VAMCs are required to follow to help ensure that RME is reprocessed correctly. In addition, VHA policy requires that VHA and VISNs oversee VAMCs' reprocessing of RME and that VAMCs report incidents involving improperly reprocessed RME.

Complexity of RME Reprocessing

According to reports from RME professional associations, the complexity of RME reprocessing has increased as the complexity of medical instruments has increased. While at one time reprocessing surgical

[18] Veterans Service Organizations provide a wide range of services for veterans and their dependents, such as assistance obtaining health care and benefits. We contacted the American Legion, Vietnam Veterans of America, and Iraq and Afghanistan Veterans of America.

and dental instruments such as scalpels and retractors might have been the bulk of a SPS program's tasks, now SPS programs are responsible for reprocessing complex instruments such as endoscopes. Reprocessing these instruments is a detailed and time-consuming process, and their increasing complexity requires a corresponding increase in the skills and time required to safely reprocess them. (See Figure 1 for an example of steps that can be required for endoscope reprocessing.)

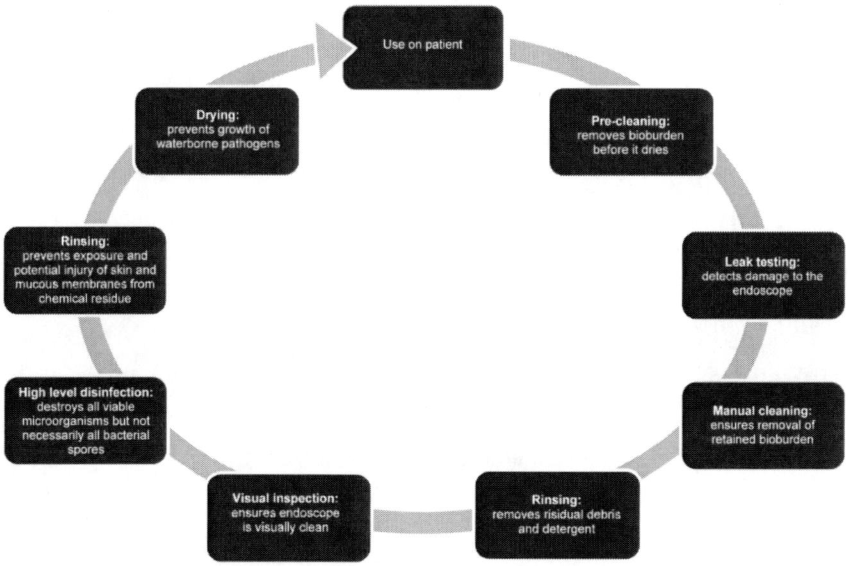

Source: GAO analysis of American Society for Gastrointestinal Endoscopy information. | GAO-18-474.

Notes: An endoscope is an instrument used for direct visual inspection of hollow organs or body cavities. Bioburden is a measure of microorganism contamination on an object. High level disinfection is performed via immersion for an appropriate duration of time in a liquid chemical germicide of appropriate concentration. According to the Association of periOperative Registered Nurses, this process is an appropriate standard of treatment for certain reusable medical equipment such as endoscopes.

Figure 1. Example of Endoscope Reprocessing Steps.

VHA Roles and Responsibilities for RME Reprocessing

Within VHA, the National Program Office for Sterile Processing under the VHA Deputy Under Secretary of Health for Operations and Management is responsible for developing RME reprocessing policies. It is also responsible for ensuring that VISNs and their respective VAMCs are adhering to its policies. Each of the 18 VISNs are responsible for ensuring adherence with VHA's RME policies at the VAMCs within its region. In turn, each of the 170 VAMCs are responsible for implementing VHA's policies related to RME. Within each VAMC, the SPS department is primarily responsible for reprocessing RME, which is used by clinicians in the operating room and other clinical service lines such as the dental and gastroenterology service. (See Figure 2.) Additionally, the SPS department collaborates with other VAMC departments such as the Environmental Management and Engineering Services on variables that affect RME reprocessing, such as the climate where RME is reprocessed.

VHA Policies for RME Reprocessing and Related Oversight

In March 2016 VHA issued Directive 1116(2)—a comprehensive policy outlining requirements for SPS programs and for overseeing RME reprocessing efforts.[19]

SPS Program Operation Requirements

To help ensure that VAMCs are reprocessing RME correctly, VHA policy establishes various requirements for the SPS programs in VAMCs

---

[19] See VHA Directive 1116(2), *Sterile Processing Services (SPS)* (March 23, 2016). This directive outlines requirements for reprocessing critical and semi-critical RME. RME is generally categorized into critical, semi-critical, or non-critical items based on the degree of risk for infection involved in use of the item. Critical items, such as surgical instruments, are those that enter sterile tissue or the vascular system and require sterilization because they confer a high risk of infection. Semi-critical items, such as certain endoscopes, are those that contact mucous membranes or non-intact skin and require only minimal high- level disinfection. Non-critical items, such as wheelchairs, are those that come into contact with intact skin and may be cleaned with low-level disinfectants. For the purposes of this report, when we refer to RME or RME policies, we are referring to critical or semi-critical RME.

to follow, such as a requirement that SPS staff monitor sterilizers to ensure that they are functioning properly, use personal protective equipment when performing reprocessing activities, separate dirty and clean RME, and maintain environmental controls. For example, VAMCs are required to maintain certain temperature, humidity, and air flow standards in areas where RME is reprocessed and stored. Additionally, in order to ensure that RME is reprocessed in accordance with manufacturers' guidelines, VAMCs are required to assess staff on their competence in following the related reprocessing steps.

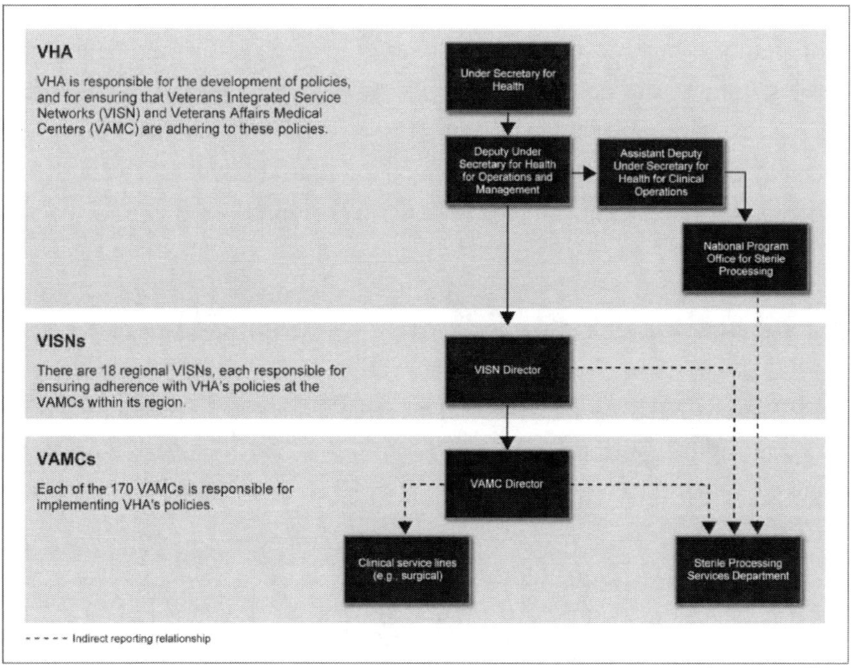

Source: GAO analysis of VHA information. | GAO-18-474.

Figure 2. Selected Veterans Health Administration (VHA) Entities' Roles and Responsibilities for Reprocessing Reusable Medical Equipment (RME).

Oversight Requirements

To help ensure that VAMCs are adhering to VHA's RME policies, VHA requires inspections, reports on incidents of improperly reprocessed RME, and corrective action plans for both non- adherent inspection results and incidents of improperly reprocessed RME.

- *Inspections.* VISNs are required to conduct annual inspections at each VAMC within their VISN and to report their inspection results to the VHA National Program Office for Sterile Processing. The VISN inspections are a key oversight tool for regularly assessing adherence to RME policies in the SPS, gastroenterology, and dental areas within VAMCs and use a standardized inspection checklist known as the SPS Inspection Tool.[20] According to VHA officials, VHA developed the SPS Inspection Tool and generally updates it annually.[21] The most recent fiscal year 2017 SPS Inspection Tool contained 148 requirements.[22] Examples of requirements include those regarding proper storage of RME and following manufacturers' instructions when reprocessing RME. Although VAMCs are also required to conduct annual self-inspections using the SPS Inspection Tool and report the results to VHA, the VISN annual inspections are a separate and important level of oversight. Finally, according to VHA officials, while not a formal policy, VHA's National Program Office for Sterile

---

[20] VISNs are also required to inspect all other clinical areas within their facility or in a community-based outpatient center in which reprocessing occurs using a separate standardized checklist known as the Clinic Inspection Tool.

[21] According to VHA officials, the SPS Inspection Tool is updated based on RME issues identified during the previous year.

[22] We considered items on the checklist to be requirements if they asked about compliance. Items that asked for descriptive information such as whether or not the VAMC had an SPS Chief were not included in our review. Of the 148 requirements, 116, 17, and 15 applied to the SPS department, gastroenterology clinic, and dental clinic, respectively. According VHA officials, there is no formal hierarchy of importance among these requirements, although for subsequent versions of the SPS Inspection Tool, VHA is considering developing a risk-based approach that will identify which requirements are the most critical.

Processing also inspects each VAMC at least once every 3 years.[23] VHA requires VISNs and VAMCs to conduct their own inspections even in years when VHA also conducts inspections.[24]

- *Incident Reports.* VHA collects incident reports or "issue briefs" generated by VAMCs on incidents involving RME to help determine the extent to which VAMCs are adhering to RME policies, among other things.[25] VHA requires VAMCs to report significant clinical incidents or outcomes involving RME that negatively affect groups or a cohort of veterans in an issue brief.[26] According to a VHA official, when VAMC staff report incidents involving RME to their facility leadership, these officials should follow VHA guidance to determine which incidents, if any, should be reported in an issue brief to the VAMC's VISN. Similarly, VISN officials, in turn, are responsible for determining whether an incident should be reported in an issue brief to VHA.
- *Corrective Action Plans.* Corrective action plans—which detail an approach for addressing any areas of policy non-adherence identified in inspections or incidents identified in issue briefs—are required at both the VISN and VAMC levels. Specifically, both VISNs and VAMCs are required to develop corrective action plans for any deficiencies identified through their inspections, and VAMCs are required to develop corrective action plans for incidents identified in issue briefs. According to a VHA official, VISNs and VAMCs are not required to send corrective action plans from inspections to VHA; however, VAMCs must send their

---

[23] In addition to the triennial inspections, VHA may conduct additional inspections for other reasons, such as at the VAMC's request or in response to concerns identified through the incident reporting process.

[24] Until the end of the first quarter of fiscal year 2017, VISNs and VAMCs were allowed to forgo their own VISN inspection if they participated in the VHA inspection of a given VAMC; in December of 2016, VHA issued a memo that required VISNs and VAMCs to perform their own inspections separately from VHA beginning in the second quarter of fiscal year 2017.

[25] These issue briefs may be related to the extent to which VAMCs are adhering to RME policies or to other RME-related issues such as plumbing malfunctions that affect RME reprocessing.

[26] See Deputy Undersecretary for Health for Operations and Management (10N), *10N Guide to VHA Issue Briefs* (June 26, 2017) and VA Directive 0321, *Serious Incident Reports* (June 6, 2012).

correction action plans to the VISN and also any related to issue briefs to VHA. Further, according to a VHA official, although neither the VAMC nor VISN corrective action plans from inspections are monitored by VHA, VHA does expect VISN officials to inform it of any critical issues that VISNs believe warrant VHA attention. For example, VHA officials would expect VISNs to report instances when RME issues result in the cancellation of procedures for multiple patients or when the VISN discovers a VAMC is lacking documentation of RME reprocessing competency assessments for a large number of their SPS staff.

Reports on Issues Related to RME Reprocessing

A number of recent reports have identified several RME-related issues at VAMCs, including non-adherence to RME policies. The issues have ranged from improperly reprocessed RME being used on patients to the cancellation of medical procedures due to lack of available RME. For example:

- In March 2018, the VA Office of Inspector General released a report describing problems identified at the Washington, D.C. VAMC, some of which were RME-related.[27] For example, the office determined that ineffective sterile processing contributed to procedure delays due to unavailable RME. The report included specific recommendations, such as ensuring there are clearly defined and effective procedures for replacing missing or broken instruments and implementing a quality assurance program to verify the cleanliness, functionality, and completeness of instrument sets before they are used in clinical areas. The VAMC Director agreed with those recommendations.

[27] Department of Veterans Affairs, Office of Inspector General, Veterans Health Administration. *Critical Deficiencies at the Washington DC VA Medical Center*. Report #17-02644-130. (Washington, D.C.: March 7, 2018.)

- In fiscal year 2017, the VA Office of Inspector General reviewed 29 VAMCs and issued reports for each in response to several RME- related complaints received through its reporting hotline.[28] The office identified issues such as staff failure to perform quality control testing on endoscopes or document their competency assessments of SPS staff in employee files. Many of the reports included specific recommendations, such as performing quality control testing on all endoscopes and ensuring SPS staff are assessed for competency at orientation and annually for the types of RME they reprocess. The VAMC Directors agreed with those recommendations.
- In 2016, the VA Office of the Medical Inspector released a report that substantiated allegations that SPS practices led to the delivery of RME with bioburden, debris, or both to the operating room.[29] The report included specific recommendations, such as reeducating SPS staff on proper SPS standards and ensuring that all training and assessments of RME reprocessing competency of SPS staff are completed as required. The VAMC Director agreed with those recommendations.
- In 2011, we released a report on VA RME that found issues with RME reprocessing. We found, for example, that VHA did not provide specific guidance on the types of RME that require device-specific training and that the guidance VHA did provide on RME reprocessing training was conflicting. We issued several recommendations for improvement, which VA has implemented.[30]

---

[28] The VA Office of Inspector General published a separate report for each of its 29 reviews. For the most recent report, see Department of Veterans Affairs Office of Inspector General, Office of Healthcare Inspections, *Clinical Assessment Program Review of the VA Eastern Colorado Health Care System, Denver, Colorado,* 16-00546-388. (Washington, D.C.: September 29, 2017). See www.va.gov/OIG/APPS/INFO/OIGOVERSIGHTREPORTS.ASPX, accessed April 9, 2018, for the remaining reports.

[29] See Department of Veterans Affairs, *Cincinnati Veterans Affairs Medical Center Cincinnati, Ohio, Veterans Integrated Service Network 10,* TRIM 2016-D-1082 (Washington, D.C.: May 8, 2016).

[30] See GAO-11-391.

VHA's Oversight Does Not Provide Reasonable Assurance that VAMCs Are Following RME Policies

VHA Does Not Have Complete Information on Adherence to RME Policies from Inspections of VAMCs

VHA has not ensured that it has complete information from the annual inspections VISNs conduct—a key oversight tool providing the most current VA-wide information on adherence to RME policies—and therefore does not have reasonable assurance that VAMCs are following RME policies intended to ensure veterans are receiving safe care.[31]

For fiscal year 2017, we determined that VHA should have had records of 144 VISN SPS inspection reports to have assurance that all required VISN SPS inspections had been conducted. However, our review shows that as of February 2018, VHA had 105 VISN SPS inspection reports and was missing 39, or more than one quarter of the required inspection reports.[32] We also determined that there were two VISNs from which VHA did not have any fiscal year 2017 reports. For the missing SPS inspection reports, VISN officials suggested several reasons why the inspections were either not conducted or conducted but the reports were not submitted to VHA. For example, officials from one of the VISNs from which VHA had

[31] Since VHA generally inspects a given VAMC once every 3 years, it relies on annual inspections led by VISNs and VAMCs for the most current VHA-wide information on the extent of adherence to RME policies. According to a VHA official, the longer a VAMC is not adhering to RME policies, the greater the risk to patient safety.

[32] There were 140 "parent" VAMCs in fiscal year 2017 for which a VISN inspection was required, and some of these VAMCs had multiple RME reprocessing locations. According to VHA officials, VHA allows VISNs to submit a single inspection report per parent VAMC, and VISNs can determine whether they want to submit separate reports if there are multiple reprocessing locations—which some did for fiscal year 2017. Until the end of the first quarter of fiscal year 2017, VISNs were allowed to forgo their own VISN inspection if they participated in the VHA inspection of a given VAMC; in December of 2016, VHA issued a memo that required VISNs to perform their own inspections separately from VHA beginning in the second quarter of fiscal year 2017. Therefore, there were a total of 144 SPS inspections reports that VHA should have had for fiscal year 2017. Even when accounting for the SPS inspections VHA was scheduled to conduct itself, there remained 21 SPS inspection reports—15 percent—which VHA did not have from either VISN or VHA inspections in fiscal year 2017. As previously noted, satellite facilities such as community-based outpatient centers or health care centers were not included in our analysis.

no SPS inspection reports told us that VISN management staffing vacancies prevented it from conducting all of its inspections.[33] An official from the other VISN from which VHA had no SPS inspection reports provided evidence that it had conducted all but one of the inspections, but the official told us the VISN did not submit reports because it has yet to receive information from VHA regarding VISN inspection outcomes, common findings, or best practices and therefore sees no value in submitting them.

VISNs provided us with evidence showing that they conducted 27 of 39 inspections that were missing from VHA's data. We analyzed these 27 reports to identify the information about non-adherence to RME policy requirements that VHA does not have from these missing VISN inspections. We determined the 10 requirements for which these VAMCs had the most non-adherence were related to quality, training, and environmental issues, among other things, with the extent of non-adherence ranging from 19 to 38 percent.[34] For example, there were 19 and 26 percent non-adherence rates to the requirements that instrument and equipment levels be sufficient to meet workloads and having a process in place to ensure staff receive make-up/repeat training, respectively. (See Appendix I.)

We also found that variation in SPS Inspection Tools and related guidance from VHA resulted in incomplete inspection results for the gastroenterology and dental areas. VHA provided VISNs with three different SPS Inspection Tools throughout the course of fiscal year 2017.[35] Although VHA guidance stated otherwise, only the third SPS Inspection

[33] The VISN provided us with evidence that it conducted one of its eight inspections but was unable to provide evidence that it had submitted them.

[34] Although we determined that VHA's summary data on the other inspections conducted by VISNs in fiscal year 2017 was not sufficiently reliable to report detailed non-adherence information, we did determine that the categories of requirements with the largest amount of non-adherence in the summary data were generally similar to those we identified among the 27 inspection reports we reviewed.

[35] VHA instructed the VISNs to continue using the fiscal year 2016 SPS Inspection Tool through December 23, 2016; the fiscal year 2017 SPS Inspection Tool through April 20, 2017; and a revised fiscal year 2017 SPS Inspection Tool beginning April 21, 2017. According to VHA officials, multiple SPS Inspection Tools have been used in prior fiscal years as well.

Tool—which was used during the second half of the fiscal year—contained requirements specific to the gastroenterology and dental areas.[36]

A VHA Central Office official told us the office hadn't been aware that it did not have all of the VISN inspection reports until it took steps to respond to our data request. The official told us VHA granted VISNs a 3-month extension for fiscal year 2017—meaning that VISNs had until the end of December 2017 to submit their inspection results—and had granted similar extensions for at least the past 4 fiscal years as well. For all of those years, the VHA official told us that the office didn't have all VISN inspection reports, even after granting extensions. As a result, VHA did not have assurance that all of the inspections had been conducted. When asked why VHA hadn't been aware that it didn't have all VISN SPS inspection reports, a VHA official said that the office has largely relied on the VISNs to ensure complete inspection result reporting because it hasn't had the resources to dedicate to monitoring inspections. The official told us that VHA has asked for and just recently received approval to hire a data analyst who could potentially be responsible for monitoring the VISN inspection reports. VHA's lack of complete information from inspection results is inconsistent with standards for internal control in the federal government regarding monitoring and information that state management should establish and operate monitoring activities and use quality information to achieve the entity's objectives.[37] Without such controls, VHA lacks reasonable assurance that VAMCs are following RME policies designed to ensure that veterans are receiving safe care.

Finally, concerns have been raised that VHA may not be receiving other important information regarding incidents of improperly reprocessed RME that, according to a VHA official, is used to update RME policy. For example, a 2016 VA Office of the Medical Inspector report found that of

---

[36] Although all three SPS Inspection Tools contained a few questions related to dental and flexible endoscopes, only the third contained an additional 15 and 17 questions specific to the dental and gastroenterology areas, respectively. According to VHA officials, VISNs were expected to use the separate Clinic Inspection Tool to inspect the dental and gastroenterology areas if not covered by one of the first two SPS Inspection Tools in fiscal year 2017; however, not all VISNs did this because VHA's guidance for all three tools stated that the dental area, gastroenterology area, or both were already covered by the SPS Inspection Tool.

[37] See GAO-14-704G.

the 22 issue briefs generated by one VAMC and sent to the VISN between fiscal years 2015 and 2016, only 7 were brought to the attention of VHA.[38] When asked about the extent to which they feel comfortable reporting incidents related to RME, almost all of the VAMC staff we spoke to said they felt comfortable doing so, although staff from two VAMCs told us they feel VAMC leadership doesn't always address or resolve reported incidents. For example, one official told us staff at their VAMC are "tired of reporting the same issues repeatedly" to facility leadership because they don't see any changes being made, but the official believes staff will continue to file reports if an incident involved a patient. All VISN officials we spoke to said they believe VAMCs are reporting significant incidents related to RME "most to all of the time." A VHA official told us they believe VHA is receiving issue briefs when necessary and that it encourages the VAMCs and VISNs to err on the side of over- rather than under-reporting; however, according to a VHA official, VHA did not require written corrective action plans for issue briefs until January 2018.[39] (See Appendix II for the percentage of issue briefs in three major categories for fiscal years 2015 through 2017.)

VHA Does Not Consistently Share Information that Could Help VAMCs Follow RME Policies

We also found that VHA does not consistently share information, particularly inspection results, with VISNs and VAMCs, and that VISNs

---

[38] According to a VHA Office of Medical Inspector official, the office determined that these issue briefs should have been forwarded from the VISN to VHA. See Department of Veterans Affairs, *Department of Veterans Affairs Cincinnati Veterans Affairs Medical Center Cincinnati, Ohio, Veterans Integrated Service Network 10,* TRIM 2016-D-1082 (Washington, D.C.: May 8, 2016).

[39] According to a VHA official, prior to January 2018, a written corrective action plan was not required for issue briefs—instead, VAMCs communicated informally with VHA. In addition to issue briefs, according to VISN and VAMC officials, VAMCs internally track incidents involving improperly reprocessed RME that do not rise to the level of requiring an issue brief, such as surgical instruments that were found to be improperly cleaned, but did not affect patient care. According to these officials, the process for reporting such incidents varies across VAMCs. For example, some VAMCs use specialized software to report, investigate, and address such incidents, while other VAMCs use less formal reporting mechanisms, such as paper-based forms.

and VAMCs would like more of this information. Specifically, about two-thirds of VISN and VAMC officials told us that sharing information on the common issues identified in the inspections of other VAMCs as well as potential solutions developed to address these issues would allow VAMCs to be proactive in strengthening their adherence to RME policies and ensuring patient safety. For example, a VAMC official told us that there were problems with equipment designed to sterilize heat- and moisture sensitive devices, and seeing how other VAMCs addressed the problem was helpful for their VAMC. Further, officials from some VISNs said VHA cited their VAMCs for issues that had been found at other facilities and, had the VAMCs been aware of the issue beforehand, they could have corrected or improved their processes earlier.

When asked about sharing inspection results and other information, VHA Central Office officials told us the office doesn't analyze or share information from VISN inspections because of a lack of resources. A VHA official told us that the office does create an internal report of common issues identified through the third of VAMCs it inspects each year, but the office doesn't share this chapter with VISNs and VAMCs because the office lacks the resources needed to prepare reports that are detailed enough to be understood correctly by recipients. According to this official, VHA has occasionally shared information it has identified on common inspection issues through newsletters, national calls, and trainings; however, VHA officials at close to half of the VISNs and VAMCs we spoke to said that they rarely or never get this information. For example, officials from one VISN told us they recall only one or two instances where VHA sent a summary of the top five RME-related issues found during inspections. Insufficient sharing of information is inconsistent with standards for internal control in the federal government regarding communication, which state that management should internally communicate the necessary quality information to achieve the entity's objectives.[40] Until this sharing becomes a regular practice, VHA is missing an opportunity to help ensure adherence to its RME policies, which are intended to ensure that veterans receive safe care.

---

[40] See GAO-14-704G.

VAMCs Report Facing Challenges Related to RME Policies and Workforce Needs, but VHA Has Not Sufficiently Addressed These Challenges

According to interviews with officials from all of the VISNs and selected VAMCs, the top five challenges VAMCs face in operating their SPS programs are related to meeting certain RME policies and challenges addressing SPS workforce needs. In particular, officials told us that VAMCs have challenges (1) meeting two RME policy requirements related to climate control monitoring and a reprocessing transportation deadline, and (2) addressing SPS workforce needs related to lengthy hiring timeframes, the need for consistent overtime, and limited pay and professional growth. (See Table 1.)

Regarding the challenges VAMCs face in meeting RME policy requirements, the majority of VISN and selected VAMC officials interviewed reported experiencing challenges adhering to two requirements from 2016 VHA issued Directive 1116(2).

- *Climate control monitoring requirement.* Officials reported that meeting the climate control monitoring requirement related to airflow and humidity is challenging for their VAMCs.[41] Under the requirement VAMCs must monitor the humidity and airflow in facility areas where RME is reprocessed and stored in order to ensure that humidity levels do not exceed a certain threshold and thereby allow the growth of microorganisms. According to almost all VISN officials, meeting the requirement is a challenge for some, if not all, of their VAMCs and in particular for older VAMCs that lack proper ventilation systems. We also found some instances of non-adherence on this issue in the group of VISN inspection reports we reviewed. In a September 2017 memorandum, VHA relaxed the requirement (e.g., adjusted the thresholds). Additionally, according to a VHA official, VHA

[41] Officials from 16 VISNs and 2 VAMCs reported experiencing challenges adhering to the airflow and humidity climate control monitoring requirement.

wants to renovate all outdated VAMC heating, ventilation, and air conditioning systems to help VAMCs meet the requirement.[42] Further, according to VHA officials, VHA also allows VAMCs to apply for a waiver exempting them from having to meet this requirement if they have an action plan in place that shows they are working toward meeting the requirement.

- *Reprocessing transportation deadline requirement.* Officials reported that meeting the reprocessing transportation deadline was also challenging for their VAMCs.[43] Under the requirement, used RME must be transported to the location where it will be reprocessed within 4 hours of use to prevent bioburden or debris from drying on the instrument and causing challenges with reprocessing. Officials reported this requirement as particularly challenging for VAMCs that must transport their RME to another facility for cleaning, such as community based outpatient clinics in rural areas that must transport their RME to their VAMC's SPS department. We also found some instances of non-adherence on this issue in the group of VISN inspection reports we reviewed. In June 2016, VHA issued a memorandum allowing the use of a pre-cleaning spray solution that, if used, allows offsite facilities such as community based outpatient clinics to transport that RME within 12 hours instead of the required 4 hours.

VHA has made some adjustments to these requirements, although some officials told us the requirements remain difficult to meet. Specifically, over half of the VISN officials reported that the climate control monitoring requirement continues to be a challenge for their VAMCs.

---

[42] VHA issued a memorandum, effective in September 2017, which updated the environmental conditions provided in VHA Directive 1116(2). The update provides interim guidance on the compliance and implementation requirements. Further, a VHA official told us that the office wants to update all HVAC systems 25 years or older still in use across the VA.

[43] Officials from 16 VISNs and two VAMCs reported experiencing challenges adhering to the reprocessing deadline requirement.

Table 1. Top Five Challenges Reported in Operating Sterile Processing Services (SPS) Programs

Challenges	**Examples provided by Veterans Integrated Service Network (VISN) and Veterans Affairs Medical Center (VAMC) Officials**
Meeting Reusable Medical Equipment (RME) Policy Requirements	
Climate control monitoring[a]	Facilities, particularly older facilities, have challenges meeting airflow and humidity requirements, especially when outside temperatures and humidity are above average.
Reprocessing transportation deadline[b]	Picking up and transporting contaminated reusable medical equipment (RME) within the deadline is a challenge, particularly for offsite clinics that must send their RME to the nearest VAMC with a SPS program.
Addressing SPS Workforce Needs	
Lengthy hiring process timeframes	It typically takes at least 3-4 months for the hiring process to be completed; as a result, VAMCs may go without SPS staff for long periods of time and lose the opportunity to hire qualified candidates.
Need for consistent overtime	Staff have to work overtime to keep up with RME workload.
Limited pay and professional growth	The limited pay and professional growth potential for SPS staff creates challenges in maintaining sufficient staff in SPS programs.

Source: GAO analysis of interviews with VISN and VAMC officials | GAO-18-474.

Note: The challenges listed in this table are results from GAO interviews with officials from the 18 VISNs and three selected VAMCs. VISN and VAMC officials outlined challenges they faced in operating their RME programs and GAO assessed which of those challenges were experienced most frequently to identify the five top challenges.

[a] Under VHA Directive 1116(2)'s climate control monitoring requirements, airflow needs to be carefully controlled in areas where RME is reprocessed and stored to minimize movement of air from dirty areas to clean areas (e.g., areas where used instruments are brought to be reprocessed and areas where unused instruments are stored before usage). Also, humidity must be monitored in the areas RME is reprocessed and stored so that humidity levels do not exceed certain thresholds.

[b] Under VHA Directive 1116(2)'s reprocessing deadline requirement, all used RME must be transported to the location where it will be reprocessed within 4 hours (or 12 hours for offsite facilities if a specific pre-cleaning spray is used, per a VHA memorandum issued on June 1, 2016).

Further, some of the officials told us that meeting the 12-hour reprocessing transportation requirement using the pre-cleaning spray was still challenging, due to the distance between clinics and their VAMC's SPS department; as a result, some facilities have decided to use disposable medical equipment that does not require reprocessing to avoid this requirement completely.[44] When we shared this information with a VHA official, the official stated that providing general information on how all facilities can meet the climate control monitoring requirement is impossible due to the uniqueness of each facility and that VHA has no further plans to adjust the reprocessing transportation deadline requirement. However, these challenges remain and some officials have expressed frustration with the limited support they've received from VHA. In September 2017 we recommended that VHA establish a mechanism by which program offices systematically obtain feedback from VISNs and VAMCs on national policy after implementation and take the appropriate actions.[45] Our findings provide further evidence of the need for VA to address this recommendation.

Regarding the challenges VAMCs face in meeting SPS workforce needs, almost all of the 18 VISN officials and officials from the three selected VAMCs reported experiencing challenges related to lengthy hiring timeframes, need for consistent overtime, and limited pay and professional growth. According to officials, these challenges result in SPS programs having difficulty maintaining sufficient staffing levels.

- *Lengthy hiring timeframes.* Officials reported that the lengthy hiring process for SPS staff creates challenges in maintaining sufficient SPS workforce.[46] For example, officials from one VISN estimated that on average it can take 3 to 4 months for a person to be hired.[47] Officials from a few other VISNs noted that not only

[44] According to the officials, using disposable medical equipment is expensive; officials from one VISN said that one VAMC spends nearly $250,000 a year on disposable medical equipment. VHA officials told us that the cost for disposable medical equipment may still be less than using RME, depending on the situation.

[45] VHA agreed with our recommendation, however, as of March 2018 had not implemented it. GAO, VA Health Care: Additional Actions Could Further Improve Policy Management, GAO-17-748 (Washington, D.C.: September 22, 2017).

[46] In our review, officials from 14 VISNs and three VAMCs reported experiencing challenges with lengthy hiring process time frames.

[47] Lengthy hiring timeframes are not unique to SPS programs at VHA. For example, in our previous report, Veterans Health Administration, *Better Data and Evaluation Could Help Improve Physician Staffing, Recruitment, and Retention Strategies*, GAO-18-124 (Washington, D.C.: October 19, 2017), we identified challenges with recruitment and hiring

does the lengthy hiring process create challenges in recruiting qualified candidates (because they accept other positions where they can be more quickly employed), but that it also results in long periods of time when SPS programs are short-staffed.

- *Need for overtime.* Officials reported that needing their SPS staff to work overtime is a challenge.[48] Specifically, 16 of the 18 VISN officials stated that there is a need for staff at their VAMCs to work overtime either "all, most, or some of the time." Further, officials from one VISN told us their VAMCs have used overtime to meet the increased workload required to implement VHA's RME policies; one official noted that the overtime has led to dissatisfaction and retention issues among SPS staff.
- *Limited pay and professional growth.* Officials identified limited pay and professional growth associated with the current pay grade as the biggest SPS workforce challenge.[49] Almost all officials stated that the current pay grade limits the pay and potential for professional growth for the two main SPS positions—medical supply technicians, who are responsible for reprocessing RME, and SPS Chiefs, who have supervisory responsibility. Specifically, the relatively low maximum allowable pay discourages staff from accepting or staying in positions and the current pay grade does not create a career path for SPS medical supply technicians to grow within the SPS department. Officials from one VISN told us that all VAMCs in their VISN have lost SPS staff due to the low pay grade for both positions. VHA officials said a proposed increase in the pay grade for SPS staff has been drafted; however, they do not know when or if it will be made effective. Further,

---

processes for physicians that caused vacancies for up to 12 months. In addition, in our previous testimony, Veterans Health Administration, *Actions Needed to Better Recruit and Retain Clinical and Administrative Staff*, GAO-17-475T (Washington, D.C.: March 22, 2017) we reported VA human resources staff experience challenges with keeping pace with work demands and that led to delays in the hiring process.

[48] In our review, officials from 16 VISNs and two VAMCs reported experiencing challenges with the need for staff to work overtime.

[49] In our review, officials from all 18 VISNs and three VAMCs reported experiencing challenges with relatively low pay. Officials from 14 VISNs and 1 VAMC reported experiencing challenges with professional growth for SPS staff.

according to officials with knowledge of the proposed changes, the changes could still be insufficient to recruit and retain SPS staff with the necessary skills and experience.

Some VISN and VAMC officials told us that difficulties maintaining sufficient SPS staff levels have in some instances adversely affected patients' access to care and increased the potential for reprocessing errors that could affect patient safety. According to these officials, staffing challenges can affect access to care when facilities have to limit or delay care—such as surgeries—because there aren't enough staff available to process all the necessary RME. An official at one VAMC told us that their SPS staff must review available RME daily to determine whether scheduled surgeries or other procedures can proceed. Further, among the 18 operating room nurse managers who responded to our inquiries, 15 indicated they have experienced operating room delays because of RME issues. In addition, some VISN and VAMC officials told us staffing challenges can potentially have an impact on patient safety, because when SPS staffing is not sufficient, mistakes are more likely to occur. For example, officials told us that if SPS staffing levels are low, particularly if they are low for an extended period of time, there is an increased chance RME will be improperly reprocessed and, if used on a patient, put that patient's safety at risk. A 2018 VA Office of Inspector General report on the Washington D.C. VAMC found that consistent SPS understaffing was a factor in SPS staff not being available to meet providers' need for reprocessed RME; according to the report, "veterans were put at risk because important supplies and instruments were not consistently available in patient care areas."[50]

While VHA is aware of these workforce challenges cited by VISN and VAMC officials, it has not studied SPS staffing at VAMCs. As a result, it does not know whether or to what extent the workforce challenges VISNs and VAMCs report adversely affect VAMCs' ability to effectively operate

---

[50] Department of Veterans Affairs, Office of Inspector General, Veterans Health Administration. *Critical Deficiencies at the Washington DC VA Medical Center.* Report #17-02644-130. (Washington, D.C.: March 7, 2018.)

their SPS programs and ensure safe care for veterans. A National Program Office of Sterile Processing official indicated that while the office might have access to some of the necessary data from VAMC SPS departments, it does not have all the necessary data or staff needed to assess SPS staffing levels.[51] Furthermore, the official added, conducting such a study would not be the responsibility of her office. Officials from the Workforce Management and Consulting Office said VHA is considering a study of SPS staffing, given the results of the VA Office of Inspector General 2018 review that identified high vacancy rates as a contributing factor to the challenges with the SPS program at the Washington D.C. VAMC. However, VHA does not have definitive plans to complete this type of study or a timeframe for when the decision will be made. Until the study is conducted and actions are taken based on the study, as appropriate, VHA will not have addressed a potential risk to its SPS programs. This is inconsistent with standards for internal control in the federal government for risk assessment, which state that management should identify, analyze, and respond to risks related to achieving defined objectives.[52] Without examining SPS workforce needs, and taking action based on this assessment, as appropriate, VHA lacks reasonable assurance that its approach to SPS staffing helps ensure veterans' access to care and safety.

CONCLUSIONS

The proper reprocessing of surgical instruments and other RME used in medical procedures is critical for ensuring veterans' access to safe care. We have previously found that VA had not provided enough guidance to

[51] In our review we found that VHA has some, but not all, of the necessary data to conduct an assessment to help determine the extent to which VAMCs have sufficient SPS staff. For example, VAMCs can collect and report to VHA data on vacancy rates and other information in an SPS staffing tool. VHA distributed a staff analysis tool for VAMCs in September 2015 and encouraged facilities to use the tool to determine the staff hours needed to operate their RME programs. Similarly, VA's National Surgery Office collects data on the number of surgical procedures cancelled due to RME issues. The surgical procedure cancellation data show that for the 12 months beginning on April 1, 2016, there were a total of 307 (or 0.8%) surgical procedures cancelled due to unavailable RME.

[52] See GAO-14-704G.

ensure SPS staff were reprocessing RME correctly; in 2016, VA issued Directive 1116(2)—with requirements for the SPS program. While this is a good step, our current review shows that VHA needs to strengthen its oversight of VAMCs' adherence to these requirements. VHA has not ensured that it has complete information from inspections of VAMCs, nor does VHA consistently share inspection results and other information that could help VAMCs meet the requirements. Without analysis of complete information from inspections and consistent sharing of this information, VHA does not have reasonable assurance that VAMCs are following all RME policies, and VHA is missing an opportunity to strengthen VAMCs' adherence to RME requirements.

Furthermore, officials from some VISNs and selected VAMCs report challenges meeting two RME policy requirements—the climate control and the reprocessing transportation deadline requirements. If VHA implements a recommendation we made in 2017 for the agency to obtain feedback from VISNs and VAMCs on their efforts to implement VHA policies and take the appropriate actions, it could help with these challenges. Additionally, while nearly all of the officials from the 18 VISNs and selected VAMCs interviewed reported challenges maintaining a sufficient SPS workforce, VHA does not know whether the current SPS workforce addresses VAMCs' SPS workforce needs. VHA officials say that VHA is considering studying its SPS workforce; however, it has not done so or announced a timeframe for doing so. Until it conducts such a study, VHA will not know whether or to what extent reported SPS workforce challenges adversely affect the ability of VAMCs to effectively operate their SPS programs and ensure access to safe care for veterans.

RECOMMENDATIONS FOR EXECUTIVE ACTION

We are making the following three recommendations to VHA:

- The Under Secretary of Health should ensure all RME inspections are being conducted and reported as required and that the inspection results VHA has are complete. (Recommendation 1)

- The Under Secretary of Health should consistently analyze and share top common RME inspection findings and possible solutions with VISNs and VAMCs. (Recommendation 2)
- The Under Secretary of Health should examine the SPS workforce needs and take action based on this assessment, as appropriate. (Recommendation 3)

AGENCY COMMENTS

We provided a draft of this chapter to VA for comment. In its written comments, which are provided in appendix III, VA concurred with our recommendations. In its comments, VA acknowledged the need for complete RME inspection information, stating that VHA will establish an oversight process for reviewing and monitoring findings from site inspections and for reporting this information to VHA leadership. Further, VA noted that VHA will analyze data from RME inspections and share findings and possible solutions with VISNs and VAMCs via a written briefing that will be published on VHA's website and discussed during educational sessions and national calls. VA also noted that VHA has an interdisciplinary work group that has identified actions it can take to address SPS workforce needs, including implementing an enhanced market-based approach for determining pay levels and developing a staffing model so VAMCs can determine what staffing levels they need to more effectively operate their SPS programs. VA expects VHA to complete all of these actions by July 2019 or earlier. As agreed with your office, unless you publicly announce the contents of this chapter earlier, we plan no further distribution until 30 days from the report date. At that time, we will send copies to the appropriate congressional committees and the Secretary of Veterans Affairs.

Sincerely yours,

Sharon Silas
Acting Director, Health Care

APPENDIX I: TOP VHA REUSABLE MEDICAL EQUIPMENT ISSUES AMONG SELECT VETERANS AFFAIRS MEDICAL CENTERS, FISCAL YEAR 2017

Table 2. Top 10 VHA Reusable Medical Equipment (RME) Policy Requirements to which Select Veterans Affairs Medical Centers (VAMC) were Non-adherent, Fiscal Year 2017

Category	Requirement	Percentage non-adherence
Quality	Demineralized water is monitored and the results are accessible to staff that reprocess RME	38
Enviro	Air pressure differential is being monitored for airflow direction in areas where RME is reprocessed	33
Quality	Random quality assurance checks are performed on instrument trays and sterile packaged items located in clean sterile storage areas	33
Training	There is a process in place to ensure staff receive make-up/repeat training	26
Enviro	A cleaning schedule or log is maintained and followed for certain cleaning	23
Training	Sterile Processing Services Level 2 certification is maintained by completing 12 continuing education units per year	22
Quality	There is use of only lint-free materials for reprocessing, storage, or protection of RME	22
Quality	The correct water is available for the final rinse cycle according to manufacturer's instructions for use	22
Admin	Instrument and equipment levels are sufficient to meet the current workload as required by stakeholders.	19
Safety	Personal Protective Equipment and work attire are provided and worn in accordance with VHA policy	19

Source: GAO analysis of Veterans Integrated Service Network data. | GAO-18-474.

Notes: This analysis was conducted using the 27 fiscal year 2017 Veterans Integrated Service Network (VISN) Sterile Processing Services (SPS) inspection reports that VHA did not have and were provided to us by the VISNs. Due primarily to the fact that some requirements weren't applicable for all 27 inspections; we chose the top10 requirements for which there was information in at least 26 of the 27 inspection reports. Denominators for the percentages in this table are therefore either 26 or 27. VHA provided VISNs with three different SPS Inspection Tools throughout the course of fiscal year 2017. The requirements included in this analysis represent those that were present in all three versions of the tools.

Our review of the 27 fiscal year 2017 inspections of VAMCs conducted by Veterans Integrated Service Networks (VISN) for which VHA did not have inspection reports identified a number of common reusable medical equipment (RME) issues among the select VAMCs. The top 10 are listed in Table 2.

APPENDIX II: PERCENTAGE OF ISSUE BRIEFS RELATED TO REUSABLE MEDICAL EQUIPMENT BY CATEGORY, FISCAL YEARS 2015-2017

Table 3. Percentage of Issue Briefs Related to Reusable Medical Equipment (RME) by Category, Fiscal Years 2015 through 2017

Category	Examples of issues in this category	Percentage of all issue briefs in this category
Process failures	Failure to follow standard operating procedures, expired items, provider misuse (e.g., improperly cleaned endoscope)	32
Physical system failures	Plumbing; heating, ventilation, and air conditioning; or sterilizer malfunction (e.g., operating room ceiling leak)	27
Physical evidence of problems	Debris or staining on reusable medical equipment (e.g., foreign objects on sterile surgical instrument tray)	19

Source: GAO analysis of VHA data. | GAO-18-474.

Notes: These percentages are out 308 total RME-related issue briefs received by the National Program Office of Sterile Processing within the Veterans Health Administration (VHA) from fiscal year 2015 through 2017. Figures do not add to 100 percent because some of the issue briefs we reviewed were administrative in nature or did not provide enough detail to categorize and are not included in this table. Administrative issue briefs are sent to VHA as a notification that the Veterans Affairs Medical Center (VAMC) has been audited by another entity such as the VA Office of Inspector General or the Joint Commission. One or more VAMC departments may be involved in problems cited in issue briefs, such as Sterile Processing Services, Environmental Management Services, and Engineering Services.

Our review of the Veterans Health Administration (VHA) summary of issue briefs for fiscal years 2015 through 2017 identified three major categories of issues related to reusable medical equipment (RME). See Table 3 for the percentage of all issue briefs that fell into each of these three categories.

APPENDIX III: COMMENTS FROM THE DEPARTMENT OF VETERANS AFFAIRS

DEPARTMENT OF VETERANS AFFAIRS
WASHINGTON DC 20420

JUL - 9 2018

Ms. Sharon Silas
Acting Director
Health Care
U.S. Government Accountability Office
441 G Street, NW
Washington, DC 20548

Dear Ms. Silas:

The Department of Veterans Affairs (VA) has reviewed the Government Accountability Office's (GAO) draft report, ***"VA HEALTH CARE: Improved Oversight Needed for Reusable Medical Equipment"*** (GAO-18-474).

The enclosure provides our general comment and sets forth the actions to be taken to address the GAO draft report recommendations.

VA appreciates the opportunity to comment on your draft report.

Sincerely,

Jacquelyn Hayes-Byrd
Acting Chief of Staff

Department of Veterans Affairs (VA) Comments to
Government Accountability Office (GAO) Draft Report
"VA HEALTH CARE: Improved Oversight Needed for Reusable Medical Equipment"
(GAO-18-474)

General Comment:

The Veterans Health Administration (VHA) is strongly committed to developing long-term solutions that mitigate risks to the timeliness, cost-effectiveness, quality and safety of the Department of Veterans Affairs (VA) health care system. We will use your findings to continue to make improvements and fulfill our mission of honoring America's Veterans by providing exceptional health care that improves their health and well-being.

The National Program Office for Sterile Processing (NPOSP) is dedicated to sustainable corrective actions. This is achieved through communication, education and training as well as commitment to collaborative policy changes with key stakeholders which include Workforce Management and Consulting, Logistics, Contracting, Facilities Management, Risk Management and Patient Safety.

As evidence of our commitment to sustainable improvements, NPOSP has implemented several actions to enhance the reporting of findings and improve communication with the field, Veterans Integrated Service Networks (VISN), and national stakeholders to provide support for success of the Sterile Processing Services (SPS) services. These actions include updating triennial action plans every 60 days, follow-up on all Issue Briefs relating to SPS, and regular calls with SPS challenged facilities. In addition, NPOSP has organized a variety of communication methods and forums to share trends. NPOSP is in the process of leading a national initiative consisting of a point in time audit, follow up training, and a VISN audit, all occurring in the next 90 days. These events will assist in establishing reliability of the SPS audit tool and ensure the NPOSP has a complete and accurate data set indicating the current performance of all SPS facilities. To assist in identifying facilities at risk, NPOSP is developing a risk assessment tool which will be available for testing in approximately 90 days.

NPOSP recognizes deficiencies and is aggressively creating cultural changes in quality improvement processes, as well as strengthening executive communication with all levels of executive leadership in order to expedite effective change and accountability.

VA is leveraging long-standing staffing models for primary care, mental health, and nursing; and is developing, evaluating, and refining additional staffing models for other functional areas. VA will continue to evolve its clinical staff modeling and workforce planning for other practice areas such as Sterile Processing.

In addition, VA is establishing a manpower capacity for the entire Department, and is committed to deploying a position management solution for both clinical and non-clinical requirements. An updated, efficiently aligned position categorization structure will enable VA facilities to more precisely define their clinical and non-clinical staffing requirements. Such a structure will also enable staffing predictive power on the part of VA medical centers and VISNs.

Recommendation 1: The Under Secretary for Health should ensure all RME inspections are being conducted and reported as required and that the inspection results VHA has are complete.

<u>VA Comment</u>: Concur. The Veterans Health Administration (VHA) National Program Office for Sterile Processing (NPOSP) will establish an oversight process for reviewing and monitoring findings from site inspections and reporting to headquarters leadership. NPOSP's oversight process will include follow-up and feedback loops with Veterans Integrated Service Networks (VISN) on their oversight of facility corrective action plans. The Office of the Deputy Under Secretary for Health for Operations and Management will ensure Sterile Processing Service (SPS) and Reusable Medical Equipment issues are reported to a current or future governance body for risk assessment and response. The target completion date reflects implementation of the new oversight and governance processes and time for data collection. The target completion date is July 2019.

<u>Recommendation 2</u>: **The Under Secretary for Health should consistently analyze and share top common RME inspection findings and possible solutions with VISNs and VAMCs.**

<u>VA Comment</u>: Concur. NPOSP will analyze data from site inspections; identify trends or risks; in collaboration with VISN, develop possible solutions; and provide a written briefing to governance, VISNs, and facilities. NPOSP will publish the briefing and possible solutions on the NPOSP website. Additionally, NPOSP will communicate the report with the VISN and VA medical center leadership through current educational sessions and national calls. The target completion date is July 2019.

<u>Recommendation 3</u>: **The Under Secretary for Health should examine the SPS workforce needs, and take action based on this assessment, as appropriate.**

<u>VA Comment</u>: Concur. VHA's Workforce Management and Consulting (WMC) is championing an interdisciplinary work group with the Office of Nursing Service (ONS), NPOSP, and the Quality, Safety and Value (QSV) High Reliability Systems and Consultation Service. The work group has identified actions to address the SPS workforce needs, including a revised qualification standard that will encompass a specified assignment for a VISN level SPS Program Manager, implementation of an enhanced market based approach to pay, and establishment of an occupational specific recruitment and development infrastructure. Additionally, WMC will provide workforce related data, as available, to assist partners in ONS, NPOSP, and QSV in their development of a staffing model for the occupation. This will allow VA medical centers

and health care systems to appropriately determine resources needs to more effectively execute mission requirements. The target completion date is December 2018.

In: Improvements Needed in the VA … ISBN: 978-1-53615-971-4
Editor: Charles Copeland

Chapter 6

IMPROVEMENTS IN OVERSIGHT NEEDED FOR REUSABLE MEDICAL EQUIPMENT*

Sharon Silas

Chairman Bergman, Ranking Member Kuster, and Members of the Subcommittee:

I am pleased to be here today to discuss the use of reusable medical equipment (RME) in the Department of Veterans Affairs (VA). As you know, VA's Veterans Health Administration (VHA) operates one of the largest health care delivery systems in the nation, serving over 9 million enrolled veterans. In providing health care services to veterans, VA medical centers use RME, such as endoscopes and surgical instruments, which must be reprocessed—that is, cleaned, disinfected, or sterilized—between uses.[1] The proper reprocessing of surgical instruments and other RME used in medical procedures is critical for ensuring veterans' access to safe care. Accordingly, VHA policy establishes requirements VA medical

---

* This is an edited, reformatted and augmented version of Testimony before the Subcommittee on Oversight and Investigations, Committee on Veterans' Affairs, House of Representatives, Publication No. GAO-18-686T, dated September 5, 2018.

[1] An endoscope is an instrument used for direct visual inspection of hollow organs or body cavities.

centers must follow when reprocessing RME to help ensure the safety of veterans who receive care at its facilities.

Nevertheless, VHA has had ongoing challenges related to properly reprocessing RME. For example, in 2011 we found that VHA had not provided sufficient guidance to VA medical center staff operating the Sterile Processing Services (SPS) programs to ensure that staff were reprocessing RME correctly, which posed potential safety risks to veterans.[2] In 2016, the VHA Office of the Medical Inspector reviewed and corroborated allegations that the SPS department at one VA medical center failed to provide surgeons with RME free of bioburden, debris, or both.[3] Further, in March 2018, the VA Office of Inspector General reported on problems at another VA medical center including delayed and cancelled procedures due to the fact that the necessary RME had not been properly reprocessed and were therefore unavailable.[4]

My testimony today summarizes the findings from our August 2018 report that analyzed VA's oversight of reusable medical equipment.[5]

Accordingly, this testimony addresses

---

[2] The VA medical center SPS programs consist of the SPS department, which has primary responsibility for reprocessing RME, and other areas such as dental clinics, where certain reprocessing functions occur. See GAO, *VA Health Care: Weaknesses in Policies and Oversight Governing Medical Supplies and Equipment Pose Risks to Veterans' Safety,* GAO-11-391 (Washington, D.C.: May 3, 2011). We recommended that VA develop and implement an approach for providing standardized training for reprocessing all critical and semi-critical RME to VA medical centers and that VA hold VA medical centers accountable for implementing device-specific training for all of these RME. VA concurred with this recommendation, and, in November 2012, stated that over 1,200 employees had been certified by a professional organization dedicated to the education and certification of SPS employees. In addition, in March 2016, VA implemented a policy which requires, among other things, standardized training for reprocessing RME and oversight of reprocessing activities.

[3] Bioburden is a measure of an object's microorganism contamination. See Department of Veterans Affairs, *Department of Veterans Affairs Cincinnati Veterans Affairs Medical Center Cincinnati, Ohio, Veterans Integrated Service Network 10,* TRIM 2016-D-1082 (Washington, D.C.: May 8, 2016).

[4] See Department of Veterans Affairs, Office of Inspector General, Veterans Health Administration, *Critical Deficiencies at the Washington DC VA Medical Center,* Report #17-02644-130 (Washington, D.C.: Mar. 7, 2018).

[5] See GAO, *VA Health Care: Improved Oversight Needed for Reusable Medical Equipment,* GAO-18-474, (Washington, D.C.: Aug. 3, 2018).

1) VHA's oversight of VA medical centers' adherence to RME policies, and
2) challenges VA medical centers face in operating their SPS programs and efforts VHA has taken to address these challenges.

As part of my testimony, I will highlight the three recommendations we made to VA to improve its oversight of RME and ensure access to safe care for veterans. VA concurred with all three of the recommendations and said it would take actions to implement them.

To conduct the work for our August 2018 report, we reviewed VHA RME policy as well as other documents such as VHA Directive 1116(2), which describes RME policy requirements and instructions for how inspections of VA medical centers' adherence to these requirements should be conducted.[6] We also reviewed VHA summary data on inspections of VA medical centers conducted by their respective Veterans Integrated Service Networks (VISN) in fiscal year 2017.[7] We reviewed the full inspection reports provided by the VISNs for inspections the VISNs had conducted in fiscal year 2017, but for which VHA did not have a record, and identified information about nonadherence to RME policy requirements. In addition, we interviewed VHA officials, officials from all 18 VISNs, and officials from four VA medical centers selected for our review.[8] As part of our review, we assessed VHA's oversight efforts and its efforts to address any identified RME-related challenges in the context

---

[6] See VHA Directive 1116(2), *Sterile Processing Services (SPS)* (Washington, D.C.: Mar. 23, 2016). See Department of Veterans Affairs, Deputy Undersecretary for Health for Operations and Management (10N), *10N Guide to VHA Issue Briefs* (Washington, D.C.: June 26, 2017).

[7] VISNs are responsible for ensuring adherence to VHA's policies among the VA medical centers within their region.

[8] We selected the four VA medical centers to achieve geographic and medical center complexity variation and the highest and lowest performance regarding operating room lag time. VHA assigns each VA medical center to one of five complexity groups based on patient population served, clinical services offered, education and research complexity, and administrative complexity. Operating room lag time data captures the time elapsed from one patient leaving and the next patient entering the operating room; lag time can be attributed to RME not being available, among other factors. The four VA medical centers we selected were located in Chicago, IL; Erie, PA; Fort Meade, SD; and Little Rock, AR. We were not able to speak with the Chief of SPS at the Chicago Jesse-Brown VA medical center; as such, some of our reported results are for three VA medical centers.

of federal standards for internal control.[9] Further details regarding the scope and methodology of our work are included in our August 2018 report. The work on which this statement is based was performed in accordance with generally accepted government auditing standards.

VHA's Oversight Does Not Provide Reasonable Assurance That VA Medical Centers Are Following RME Policies

In our August 2018 report, we found that VHA had not ensured that it has complete information from the annual inspections VISNs conduct. VISNs are required to conduct annual inspections at each VA medical center within their VISN and to report their inspection results to VHA. These inspections are a key oversight tool providing the most current information on adherence to RME policies VA-wide, as VHA does not inspect every VA medical center each year. VHA's lack of complete information from inspection results is inconsistent with standards for internal control in the federal government regarding monitoring and information that state management should establish and operate monitoring activities and use quality information to achieve the entity's objective.[10] Without complete information from these inspections, VHA cannot reasonably ensure that VA medical centers are following RME policies intended to ensure veterans are receiving safe care.

For fiscal year 2017, we determined that VHA was missing 39—or more than one-quarter—of the required VISN inspection reports.[11] VISN officials suggested several reasons for the missing reports. For example, an official from one VISN provided evidence that the VISN had conducted

---

[9] See GAO, Standards for Internal Control in the Federal Government, GAO-14-704G (Washington, D.C.: September 2014). Internal control is a process effected by an entity's oversight body, management, and other personnel that provides reasonable assurance that the objectives of an entity will be achieved.

[10] See GAO-14-704G.

[11] VISNs were able to provide GAO with evidence that they had conducted 27 of the 39 missing inspections.

almost all of its inspections, but told us the VISN did not submit reports to VHA because it has yet to receive information from VHA regarding VISN inspection outcomes, common findings across VISNs, or best practices and therefore the VISN sees no value in submitting the reports. A VHA official told us the office had not been aware that it did not have all of the required VISN inspection reports because it has largely relied on the VISNs to monitor inspections since VHA does not have sufficient resources to do so itself.

We also found in our report that VHA does not consistently share information, particularly inspection results, with VISNs and VA medical centers, and that VISNs and VA medical centers would like more of this information. Specifically, about two-thirds of the VISN and VA medical center officials we interviewed told us that sharing information on the common issues identified by VA medical center inspections as well as potential solutions developed to address these issues would allow the VA medical centers to be proactive in strengthening their adherence to RME policies and ensuring patient safety. For example, one VA medical center official we interviewed told us that there were problems with equipment designed to sterilize heat- and moisture- sensitive devices, and that seeing how other VA medical centers addressed the problem would be helpful. Further, officials from some VISNs we interviewed said VHA cited their VA medical centers for issues that had been found at other facilities and that, had they been aware of the issue beforehand, they could have corrected or improved their processes for adhering to RME policies.

When asked about sharing inspection results and other information, VHA Central Office officials told us the office does not analyze or share VISN inspections information due to inadequate resources. More specifically, one VHA official told us that the office does create an internal report of common issues identified through the third of VA medical centers it inspects each year, but does not share this chapter with VISNs and VA medical centers because the office lacks the resources needed to prepare reports that are detailed enough to be correctly understood by the VISN and VA medical center recipients. According to this official, VHA has occasionally shared information regarding common inspection issues through newsletters, national calls, and trainings. However, VHA officials we interviewed at 8 of the 18 VISNs and 1 of the 4 VA medical centers we reviewed said that they rarely or never received such information. For example, officials from one VISN told us that they recall just one or two instances where VHA sent a summary of the top five RME-related issues found during VHA inspections. Insufficient sharing of information is inconsistent with standards for internal control in the federal government regarding communication, which state that management should internally communicate the necessary quality information to achieve the entity's objectives.[12] Until this sharing becomes a regular practice, VHA is missing an opportunity to help ensure adherence to its RME policies, which are intended to ensure that veterans receive safe care.

Based on our findings, in our August 2018 report we recommended that VA take steps to ensure that all RME inspections are being conducted and the results of those inspections are reported to VHA as required. We also recommended that VA consistently analyze and share top common RME inspection findings and possible solutions with VISNs and VA medical centers. VA concurred with these recommendations and said it would establish an oversight process for reviewing and monitoring findings from RME inspections and for reporting this information to VHA leadership. Further, VA noted that VHA will analyze data from RME inspections and share findings and possible solutions with VISNs and VA medical centers via a written briefing.

VA Medical Centers Reported Facing Challenges Related to RME Policies and Workforce Needs, but VHA Has Not Sufficiently Addressed These Challenges

We also found in our August 2018 report that the top challenges VA medical centers face in operating their SPS programs were related to

[12] See GAO-14-704G.

meeting certain RME policy requirements and challenges addressing SPS workforce needs. Regarding the challenges VA medical centers face in meeting RME policy requirements, the majority of the 18 VISN and four selected VA medical center officials interviewed reported experiencing challenges adhering to two requirements from VHA's 2016 Directive 1116(2).

- Climate control monitoring requirement. According to officials from 16 VISNs and two VA medical centers, meeting the climate control monitoring requirement related to humidity and airflow in facility areas where RME is reprocessed and stored is a challenge for some, if not all, of their VA medical centers, particularly older VA medical centers that lack proper ventilation systems.[13]
- Reprocessing transportation deadline requirement. Officials from 16 VISNs and two VA medical centers reported that meeting the reprocessing transportation deadline was challenging for their VA medical centers. They said this was particularly challenging for VA medical centers that must transport their RME to another facility for cleaning, such as community based outpatient clinics in rural areas that must transport their RME to their VA medical center's SPS department.[14] Under the requirement, used RME must be transported to the location where it will be reprocessed within 4 hours of use to prevent bioburden or debris from drying on the instrument and causing reprocessing challenges.

In a report we issued in September 2017 examining VA's policy management practices, we recommended that VHA establish a mechanism

---

[13] Under the climate control monitoring requirement, airflow needs to be carefully controlled in areas where RME is reprocessed and stored to minimize movement of air from dirty areas to clean areas (e.g., areas where used instruments are brought to be reprocessed and areas where unused instruments are stored before usage). Also, humidity must be monitored in the areas RME is reprocessed and stored so that humidity levels do not exceed certain thresholds.

[14] Under the reprocessing deadline requirement, all used RME must be transported to the location where it will be reprocessed within 4 hours (or 12 hours for offsite facilities if a specific pre-cleaning spray is used, per a VHA memorandum issued on June 1, 2016).

through which program offices could systematically obtain feedback from VISN and VA medical center officials after the implementation of new national policies.[15] The more recent findings of our August 2018 report provide further evidence of the need for VA to address that recommendation.

Regarding the challenges VA medical centers face in meeting SPS workforce needs, almost all of the 18 VISN officials and officials from the three selected VA medical centers we interviewed reported experiencing challenges related to lengthy hiring timeframes, the need for consistent overtime practices, and limited pay and opportunities for professional growth. According to these officials, such challenges make it difficult for SPS programs to maintain sufficient staffing levels.

- Lengthy hiring timeframes. Officials from 14 VISNs and three VA medical centers reported that the lengthy hiring process for SPS staff creates challenges in maintaining a sufficient SPS workforce. For example, officials from one VISN estimated that it can take 3 to 4 months on average to hire a new SPS staff member.
- Need for overtime. Officials from 16 VISNs and two VA medical centers reported that needing SPS staff to work overtime is a challenge. Further, officials from one VISN told us that their VA medical center had used overtime to meet increased workload demands required to implement VHA's RME policies. One official we interviewed noted that the overtime has led to dissatisfaction and retention issues among SPS staff.
- Limited pay and opportunities for professional growth. Officials identified limited pay and lack of opportunities for professional growth as the biggest SPS workforce challenge.[16] These officials stated that the relatively low maximum allowable pay discourages

---

[15] VHA agreed with our recommendation; however, as of March 2018 VHA had not implemented it. GAO, *VA Health Care: Additional Actions Could Further Improve Policy Management,* GAO-17-748 (Washington, D.C.: Sept. 22, 2017).

[16] In our review, officials from all 18 VISNs and three VA medical centers reported experiencing challenges with relatively low pay. Officials from 14 VISNs and 1 VA medical center reported experiencing challenges with professional growth for SPS staff.

staff from accepting or staying in SPS positions and the current pay grade does not create a career path for SPS medical supply technicians to grow within the SPS department. VHA officials told us that a proposed increase in the pay grade for SPS staff has been drafted; however, the officials do not know when or if it will be made effective. Further, according to VHA officials with knowledge of the proposed changes, the changes could still be insufficient to recruit and retain SPS staff with the necessary skills and experience.

While VHA is aware of these workforce challenges cited by VISN and VA medical center officials, it has not studied SPS staffing issues at VA medical centers. VHA officials told us that VHA is considering studying its SPS workforce. However, the agency has not announced a plan or a timeframe for doing so. Until the study is conducted and actions are taken based on the study, as appropriate, VHA will not have addressed a potential risk to its SPS programs. This is inconsistent with standards for internal control in the federal government for risk assessment, which state that management should identify, analyze, and respond to risks related to achieving defined objectives.[17] Without examining SPS workforce needs, and taking action based on this assessment, as appropriate, VHA lacks reasonable assurance that its approach to SPS staffing helps ensure veterans' access to care and safety.

Based on our findings, we recommended in our August 2018 report that VA assess its SPS workforce needs, and take action based on this assessment, as appropriate. VA concurred with this recommendation and said that VHA has an interdisciplinary work group that has identified actions it can take to address SPS workforce needs.

Chairman Bergman, Ranking Member Kuster, and Members of the Subcommittee, this concludes my statement. I would be pleased to respond to any questions that you may have at this time.

---

[17] See GAO-14-704G.

In: Improvements Needed in the VA … ISBN: 978-1-53615-971-4
Editor: Charles Copeland

Chapter 7

VA HEALTH CARE: IMPROVED GUIDANCE AND OVERSIGHT NEEDED FOR THE PATIENT ADVOCACY PROGRAM*

United States Government Accountability Office

ABBREVIATIONS

CARA	Comprehensive Addiction and Recovery Act of 2016
FY	fiscal year
OIG	Office of Inspector General
OPA	Office of Patient Advocacy
OPCC&CT	Office of Patient Centered Care and Cultural Transformation
PATS	Patient Advocate Tracking System
ROC	report of contact
VA	Department of Veterans Affairs
VAMC	VA medical center

* This is an edited, reformatted and augmented version of United States Government Accountability Office, Report to Congressional Committees, Publication No. GAO-18-356, dated April 2018.

VHA	Veterans Health Administration
VISN	Veterans Integrated Service Network
VSO	veterans service organization.

WHY GAO DID THIS STUDY

VHA has designated patient advocates at each VAMC to receive and document feedback from veterans or their representatives, including requests for information, compliments, and complaints. In recent years, the importance of a strong patient advocacy program has taaken on new significance given concerns with VHA's ability to provide veterans timely access to health care, among other issues.

The Comprehensive Addiction and Recovery Act of 2016 included a provision for GAO to review VHA's patient advocacy program. This chapter examines the extent to which VHA has (1) provided guidance on the governance of the program; (2) provided guidance on staffing the program; (3) assessed the training needs of patient advocates and monitored training completion; and (4) monitored patient advocacy program data-entry practices and reviewed program data. GAO reviewed VHA and VAMC documents, including summaries of program data. GAO interviewed VHA officials about the program, as well as officials from a non-generalizable selection of eight VAMCs and five VISNs selected based on the volume of veteran complaints and other factors. GAO also compared VHA policies and practices to federal internal control standards.

WHAT GAO RECOMMENDS

GAO is making 6 recommendations to improve guidance for and oversight of the patient advocacy program, focusing on governance, staffing, training, and PATS data entry and assessment. VA concurred with GAO's recommendations.

What GAO Found

The Veterans Health Administration (VHA) provided limited guidance to Department of Veterans Affairs (VA) medical centers (VAMC) on the governance of its patient advocacy program and its guidance, a program handbook, has been outdated since 2010. VAMCs are still expected to follow the outdated handbook, which does not provide needed details on governance, such as specifying the VAMC department to which patient advocates should report. Officials from most of the VAMCs that GAO reviewed noted that the VAMC department to which patient advocates report can have a direct effect on the ability of staff to resolve veterans' complaints. The lack of updated and complete guidance may impede the patient advocacy program from meeting its expectations, to receive and address complaints from veterans in a convenient and timely manner.

VHA also has provided limited guidance to VAMCs on staffing the patient advocacy program. VHA's handbook states that every VAMC should have at least one patient advocate and appropriate support staff; however, it did not provide guidance on how to determine the number and type of staff needed. Officials at all but one of the eight VAMCs in GAO's review stated that their patient advocacy program staff had more work to do than they could accomplish. This limited guidance on staffing could impede VAMCs' efforts to ensure that they have the appropriate number and type of staff to address veterans' complaints in a timely manner.

Further, VHA has recommended training for patient advocates, but it has not developed an approach to routinely assess their training needs or monitored training completion. VHA officials stated that they relied on VAMC and Veterans Integrated Service Network (VISN) staff to conduct these activities. However, GAO found that for the eight VAMCs in its review, the training needs of patient advocates were not routinely assessed, and training completion was not always monitored. Without conducting these activities, VHA increases its risk that staff may not be adequately trained to advocate on behalf of veterans.

Finally, VHA has not monitored patient advocacy program data-entry practices or reviewed the data to assess program performance. VHA officials stated that they relied on VISN and VAMC officials to ensure that all complaints were consistently entered into VHA's Patient Advocate Tracking System (PATS). However, GAO identified inconsistencies in the extent to which VAMC officials did so. VHA's lack of monitoring may pose a risk that not all complaints are entered into this tracking system—a goal of the program. Additionally, VHA officials stated they did not systemically review data in the system to assess program performance and identify potential system-wide improvements because VHA considered this the responsibility of VAMCs. As a result, VHA officials may miss opportunities to improve veterans' experiences.

VHA is beginning to address many of these governance, staffing, training, and data issues, including directing a workgroup to provide recommendations by spring of 2018. However, because the recommendations will be advisory, and because program deadlines have slipped in the past, the nature and timing of the actions needed to resolve these issues remain unclear.

April 12, 2018

The Honorable Johnny Isakson
Chairman

The Honorable Jon Tester
Ranking Member
Committee on Veterans' Affairs
United States Senate

The Honorable Phil Roe, MD
Chairman

The Honorable Tim Walz
Ranking Member
Committee on Veterans' Affairs
House of Representatives

The Veterans Health Administration (VHA), within the Department of Veterans Affairs (VA), operates one of the nation's largest health care systems. VA has faced a growing demand by veterans for its health care services due, in part, to (1) servicemembers returning from the United States' military operations in Afghanistan and Iraq and (2) the growing needs of an aging veteran population—trends that are expected to continue. The total number of veteran enrollees in VA's health care system rose from 7.9 million to almost 9 million from fiscal year (FY) 2006 through FY 2016. As the number of veterans using VA health care services increases, it is important to ensure that feedback about their care is addressed in a convenient and timely manner. To that end, VHA has designated patient advocates at each VA medical center (VAMC) to receive and document feedback from veterans or their representatives, including requests for information, compliments, and complaints.[1]

Although VHA's patient advocacy program has been in place since 1990, it has taken on new significance in recent years given concerns about veterans' ability to receive timely and quality care, among other issues. Our work, along with that of the VA Office of Inspector General (OIG) and others, has cited longstanding concerns about VA's oversight of its health care system, including ambiguous policies and inconsistent processes.[2] These concerns contributed to the addition of veterans' health care to GAO's High-Risk List in 2015, and its continued inclusion in the 2017 update.[3] In 2017, the VA OIG raised concerns about the effectiveness

---

[1] In this report, the term "VAMC" refers to an individual VA medical center and any of its associated facilities such as community-based outpatient clinics.

[2] For example, see GAO, *Veterans Health Care: Additional Actions Could Further Improve Policy Management*, GAO-17-748 (Washington, D.C.: Sept. 22, 2017), and *VA Health Care: Improved Policies and Oversight Needed for Reviewing and Reporting Providers for Quality and Safety Concerns*, GAO-18-63 (Washington, D.C., Nov. 15, 2017). See also, for example, Department of Veterans Affairs, Office of Inspector General, *Veterans Health Administration, Review of the Implementation of the Veterans Choice Program*, Report No. 15-04673-333 (Washington, D.C.: Jan. 30, 2017), and *Veterans Health Administration, Audit of Veteran Wait Time Data, Choice Access, and Consult Management in VISN 6*, Report No. 16-02618-424 (Washington, D.C.: Mar. 2, 2017).

[3] GAO maintains a high-risk list to focus attention on government agencies and programs that it identifies as high risk due to their greater vulnerabilities to fraud, waste, abuse, and mismanagement or the need for transformation to address economy, efficiency, or effectiveness challenges. See GAO, *High-Risk Series: An Update,* GAO-15-290 (Washington, D.C.: Feb. 11, 2015). In our 2017 high-risk update, we reported that

of VHA's patient advocacy program, including a lack of monitoring of program data, such as feedback documented by advocates, to identify trends across VAMCs.[4]

Until recently, VHA's patient advocacy program was overseen by the Office of Patient Centered Care and Cultural Transformation (OPCC&CT). However, the Comprehensive Addiction and Recovery Act of 2016 (CARA), included a provision for VHA to establish an Office of Patient Advocacy (OPA) by July 2017 to take on oversight responsibilities for the program, such as ensuring that patient advocates at VAMCs receive training.[5]

CARA also included a provision for us to review VHA's patient advocacy program.[6] This chapter examines the extent to which VHA has

1. provided guidance to VAMCs on the governance of the program;
2. provided guidance to VAMCs on staffing the program;
3. assessed the training needs of patient advocates and monitored training completion; and
4. monitored patient advocacy program data-entry practices and reviewed program data.

For all four objectives, we interviewed officials involved in the patient advocacy program from eight VAMCs and their five associated Veterans Integrated Service Networks (VISN), regional networks of care. We selected six of our eight VAMCs for variation in (1) the number of complaints received and entered in VHA's Patient Advocate Tracking System (PATS)—an electronic system used to describe and track the resolution of veterans' feedback across VAMCs—in FY 2016, (2) facility

---

previously identified issues for policy management continue, in part, because VA lacks the capacity to effectively address the issues we raised. See GAO, *High-Risk Series: Progress on Many High-Risk Areas, While Substantial Efforts Needed on Others*, GAO-17-317 (Washington D.C.: Feb. 15, 2017).

[4] Department of Veterans Affairs, Office of Inspector General, *Veterans Health Administration, Audit of the Patient Advocacy Program*, Report No. 15-05379-146. (Washington, D.C.: Mar. 31, 2017).

[5] Comprehensive Addiction and Recovery Act of 2016, Pub. L. No. 114-198, § 924, 130 Stat. 695, 767-769 (2016).

[6] Pub. L. No. 114-198, § 923, 130 Stat. 695, 767 (2016).

complexity level, (3) geographic location, and (4) the type of staff VAMCs used to administer the program.[7] We selected the remaining two VAMCs based on one's involvement in piloting a new approach to recording patient advocacy program data, and one's recent changes to the structure of its program. We also ensured that at least three of the VAMCs we selected received assessments from OPCC&CT on how they had implemented the patient advocacy program to gain perspectives on the office's involvement with VAMCs.[8] See Table 1 for a list of the eight VAMCs we selected and their associated VISNs. Perspectives obtained from the eight VAMCs and five VISNs in our review cannot be generalized.

Table 1. Selected Department of Veterans Affairs Medical Centers (VAMC) and Associated Veterans Integrated Service Networks (VISN) Included in Review

VAMC	VISN
Edith Nourse Rogers Memorial Veterans Hospital (Bedford, Massachusetts)	1
VA Maryland Health Care System (Baltimore, Maryland)	5
Fayetteville VA Medical Center (Fayetteville, North Carolina)	6
Hampton VA Medical Center (Hampton, Virginia)	6
John J. Pershing VA Medical Center (Poplar Bluff, Missouri)	15
Kansas City VA Medical Center (Kansas City, Missouri)	15
Grand Junction Veterans Health Care System (Grand Junction, Colorado)	19
VA Eastern Colorado Health Care System (Denver, Colorado)	19

Source: GAO analysis of Veterans Health Administration (VHA) information. | GAO-18-356.

We also interviewed VHA officials, including those who had overseen the program when it was under OPCC&CT and who transitioned to OPA once the office was established in 2017. In addition, we interviewed officials from five veterans service organizations (VSO) to obtain their

[7] VHA categorizes VAMCs according to complexity level, which is determined on the basis of the characteristics of the patient population, clinical services offered, educational and research missions, and administrative complexity. We obtained the number of complaints received by VAMCs and recorded in PATS in FY 2016 from VISN officials in March 2017. We then ranked VAMCs by the number of complaints and split them into three equal groups. We then selected at least two VAMCs from each of these groups.

[8] In 2015 and 2016, OPCC&CT conducted assessments of the implementation of the patient advocacy program at some VAMCs and provided recommendations on how to strengthen program implementation to better align with a proactive approach to patient advocacy.

perspectives on the patient advocacy program: American Legion, Disabled American Veterans, Iraq and Afghanistan Veterans of America, Veterans of Foreign Wars, and Vietnam Veterans of America.[9]

To examine the extent to which VHA has provided guidance to VAMCs on the governance of the patient advocacy program, we reviewed VHA's handbook for the program to determine, among other things, whether it specified the VAMC department to which patient advocates should report and whether it identifies responsibilities for VHA staff overseeing the program.[10] We also reviewed documentation of VHA's planned efforts related to improving the governance of the program, such as a draft directive for the program. We evaluated the information we reviewed in VHA's handbook against federal internal control standards.[11]

To examine the extent to which VHA has provided guidance to VAMCs on staffing the patient advocacy program, we reviewed VHA's handbook for the program. Specifically, we reviewed the handbook to determine the extent to which it provided guidance on how VAMCs should determine the appropriate number and type of staff needed to administer the program. We also reviewed documentation of VHA's planned efforts related to staffing the program identified in a workgroup charter. We evaluated VHA's efforts to provide guidance to VAMCs on staffing against key principles for effective strategic workforce planning and federal internal control standards.[12]

To examine the extent to which VHA has assessed the training needs of patient advocates and monitored training completion, we reviewed training materials VHA provided to VAMCs, such as a list of recommended training for patient advocates. We also reviewed documentation of VHA's planned efforts related to assessing the training

---

[9] We selected five VSOs based on several criteria including whether the organization published articles or reports about VHA's patient advocacy program.

[10] For example, see Department of Veterans Affairs, *Veterans Health Administration*, *VHA Patient Advocacy Program,* VHA Handbook 1003.4 (Sept. 2, 2005).

[11] GAO, *Standards for Internal Control in the Federal Government,* GAO-14-704G (Washington, D.C.: September 2014). Internal control is a process effected by an entity's oversight body, management, and other personnel that provides reasonable assurance that the objectives of an entity will be achieved.

[12] See GAO-14-704G and GAO *Human Capital: Key Principles for Effective Strategic Workforce Planning,* GAO-04-39 (Washington, D.C.: Dec. 11, 2003).

needs of patient advocates identified in a workgroup charter. We evaluated the extent to which VHA has monitored training of patient advocates against a guide for assessing strategic training and development efforts and federal internal control standards.[13]

To examine the extent to which VHA has monitored data-entry practices and reviewed data from the patient advocacy program, we reviewed VHA's handbook for the program and summaries of data from PATS.[14] We also reviewed documentation of VHA's planned efforts related to PATS data-entry practices and reviewing program data identified in a workgroup charter. We evaluated the extent to which VHA has monitored data-entry practices and reviewed PATS data against a guide for assessing the reliability of computer-processed data and federal internal control standards.[15]

We conducted this performance audit from February 2017 to April 2018 in accordance with generally accepted government auditing standards. Those standards require that we plan and perform the audit to obtain sufficient, appropriate evidence to provide a reasonable basis for our findings and conclusions based on our audit objectives. We believe that the evidence obtained provides a reasonable basis for our findings and conclusions based on our audit objectives.

BACKGROUND

VHA's patient advocacy program is intended to provide veterans with a means to provide feedback about health care services they receive at VAMCs. VHA sets forth minimum expectations for VAMCs' administration of the program, including that veterans must have easy

---

[13] See GAO-14-704G and GAO, *Human Capital: A Guide for Assessing Strategic Training and Development Efforts in the Federal Government*, GAO-04-546G (Washington, D.C.: Mar. 1, 2004).

[14] To obtain contextual information related to the patient advocacy program, we reviewed VA analyses of data for fiscal years 2014 through 2017 that had been entered in PATS as of January 4, 2018.

[15] See GAO-14-704G and GAO, *Assessing the Reliability of Computer-Processed Data,* GAO-09-680G (Washington, D.C.: July 2009).

access to a patient advocate and must have their complaints addressed in a convenient and timely manner.

Administration of the Patient Advocacy Program

The patient advocacy program is administered at the VAMC level. Each of VA's 170 VAMCs is responsible for making at least one patient advocate available to respond to veterans' feedback, and for ensuring that feedback is recorded in PATS. VAMCs may designate other staff to assist patient advocates in responding to feedback, such as lead patient advocates and service-level advocates. Service-level advocates, such as nurses or administrative staff, are designated at some VAMCs to respond to veterans' feedback before involving a patient advocate. All VAMC staff that have a designated role in the administration of the patient advocacy program are referred to as patient advocacy program staff. In addition to designating program staff, VAMCs may use a variety of methods to make veterans aware of the patient advocacy program, such as displaying signage on site and including information about the program on their websites. (See app. I for more information on the methods selected VAMCs used to make veterans aware of the program).

Patient advocacy program staff enter veterans' feedback in PATS using a report of contact (ROC) and assign one or more issue codes that generally describe the nature of the feedback, such as coordination of care. (See app. II for additional information on entering veterans' feedback into PATS.) Each piece of feedback shared is categorized as either a request for information, compliment, or complaint. VHA's handbook for the program specifies certain goals for data collection and resolution—specifically, that

- all complaints should be entered in PATS to enable a comprehensive understanding of veterans' issues and concerns to, in turn, identify potential system-wide improvements; and

- responses should occur no later than 7 days after the complaint is made.[16]

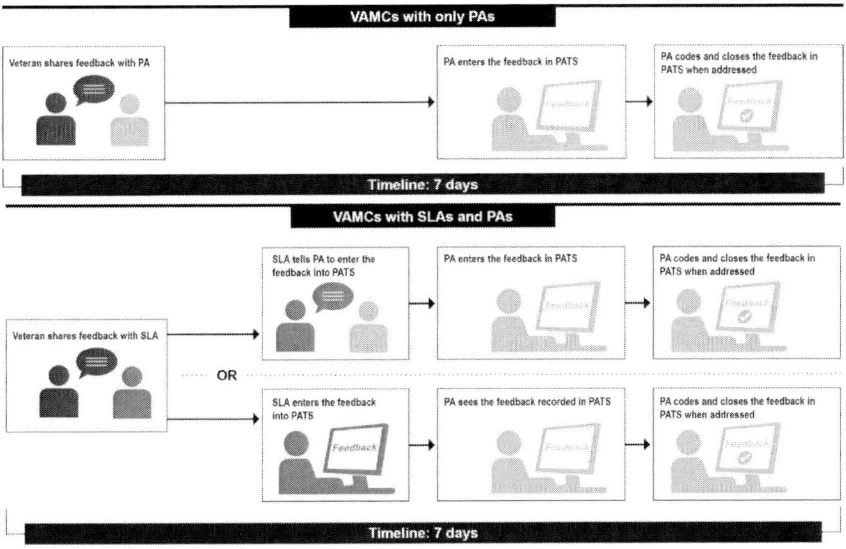

Legend: PA= patient advocate; PATS= Patient Advocate Tracking System; SLA= service-level advocate; VAMC= Department of Veterans Affairs Medical Center.

Source: GAO analysis of Veterans Health Administration (VHA) documents and interviews with VHA officials. | GAO-18-356.

Note: In this figure the term "veteran" includes veterans and their representatives, such as family members or friends, and the term "feedback" includes requests for information, compliments, and complaints. Patient advocates are VHA employees designated at each VAMC to receive feedback from veterans. Service-level advocates, such as nurses or administrative staff, are designated at some VAMCs to receive veterans' feedback before involving a patient advocate. According to VHA's handbook for the program, responses to complaints should occur as soon as possible, but no longer than 7 days after the complaint is made. VHA officials told us they interpret this goal to mean that complaints should be closed in PATS within 7 days. Other forms of feedback (requests for information and compliments) are not required to be entered in PATS but may be entered, as this information is useful in determining common areas of confusion that could be addressed in a proactive manner.

Figure 1. Process at Department of Veterans Affairs Medical Centers (VAMC) for Entering and Closing Veterans' Feedback in the Patient Advocate Tracking System.

---

[16] See VHA Handbook 1003.4.

With this guidance, patient advocacy program staff use a variety of approaches for entering veterans' feedback in PATS and closing it in the system once addressed. For example, when VAMCs have designated service-level advocates, the process for entering and closing feedback in PATS is generally different than the approach used by VAMCs that have only patient advocates (See Figure 1).

Oversight of the Patient Advocacy Program

Patient advocacy program staff at each VAMC are assisted by a VISN-level coordinator who acts as a liaison between the VAMCs and VHA and is responsible for ensuring consistency in PATS data collection within the VISN. The VISN director is responsible for designating the coordinator and ensuring that each VAMC within the VISN has at least one patient advocate.

The VHA office responsible for overseeing the patient advocacy program changed as a result of CARA. From January 2011 to July 2017, the program was overseen by OPCC&CT under VHA's Deputy Under Secretary for Health for Operations & Management.[17] CARA included a provision for VHA to establish OPA to begin overseeing the program and specified that this office would report directly to the Under Secretary for Health, a higher-level office within VHA.[18] Although OPCC&CT is no longer responsible for overseeing the program, it is to continue to play an advisory role to OPA during the initial phases of its work, according to OPCC&CT officials.

Many of OPA's oversight responsibilities are specified in CARA including ensuring that patient advocates advocate on behalf of veterans, manage PATS, and identify trends in the data to determine whether there are opportunities for improving veterans' health care. Also, OPA's director is required to ensure that patient advocates receive relevant, consistent

[17] VHA's patient advocacy program was established in 1990. From the program's inception to January 2011, the program was overseen by the National Veteran Service and Advocacy Program of the VISN Support Service Center.

[18] Pub. L. No. 114-198, § 924, 130 Stat. 767 (2016), codified at 38 U.S.C. §7309A(c)(2)(C)

training across VAMCs. When establishing the office in July 2017, VHA officials wrote a memo indicating that OPA's primary objectives were to implement a standardized policy for the patient advocacy program and to resolve any system-wide issues, such as concerns about care across VAMCs identified through veterans' feedback. In addition, in August 2017, OPA began soliciting feedback from VAMCs on various aspects of the patient advocacy program to identify improvement priorities and best practices. By September 2017, OPA had identified an acting program director, established a workgroup (called the National Strategic Workgroup) to develop recommendations related to program administration, and finalized a charter that identifies workgroup deliverables.

VHA Has Provided Limited, Outdated Guidance to VAMCs on the Governance of the Patient Advocacy Program

VHA has provided limited guidance to VAMCs on the governance of the patient advocacy program. Specifically, VHA provided limited guidance on how to meet the program's expectations that veterans have easy access to a patient advocate who will hear their complaints and address them in a timely manner. While VHA's handbook for the program provides general information on the responsibilities of patient advocacy program staff, it does not specify the VAMC department to which patient advocates should report to help ensure VAMCs meet these expectations. According to VHA officials, the lack of specific guidance was intentional and due in part to VHA officials' view that leadership at each VAMC is in the best position to understand the needs of veterans at their facilities, and therefore should have flexibility to make decisions about governance in response to those needs.

In addition to providing limited guidance to VAMCs, VHA's patient advocacy program handbook is out of date and does not incorporate recent agency-wide changes, such as those made in response to *VHA Strategic*

Plan FY 2013 – 2018 which identifies the goal of providing proactive, patient-driven health care.[19] The handbook for the program was issued in 2005, expired in 2010, and as of January 2018, no updates had been released. In the absence of an updated document, VAMCs are still expected to follow the outdated handbook.[20] However, the handbook does not identify the responsibilities of the current VHA office responsible for overseeing the program. Instead, it identifies the responsibilities of the VHA office that oversaw the program before OPCC&CT began overseeing the program in 2011.

In recent years, OPCC&CT reviewed the implementation of the patient advocacy program at some VAMCs and provided specific recommendations on how to change program governance to better reflect a more proactive patient advocacy program model. However, the recommendations from these reviews were provided only to some VAMCs; guidance that could be applicable to all VAMCs was not added to the handbook.[21] OPCC&CT officials stated that they did not update the handbook because they decided to instead spend time trying to understand recent feedback they received from VAMC officials and ensure that any updates would reflect system-wide shifts as a result of VHA's strategic plan.

OPCC&CT's limited and outdated guidance to VAMCs on the governance of the patient advocacy program is inconsistent with federal internal control standards for the control environment, which require agencies to establish an organizational structure, assign responsibility, and delegate authority to achieve agency objectives—key aspects of

---

[19] See Department of Veterans Affairs, Veterans Health Administration, *VHA Strategic Plan FY 2013 – 2018*.

[20] See Department of Veterans Affairs, Veterans Health Administration, *Controlled National Policy/Directives Management System*, VHA Directive 6330 (Washington, D.C.: June 24, 2016).

[21] According to an assessment OPCC&CT completed for one VAMC on the implementation of the patient advocacy program, for example, in a proactive model of the patient advocacy program, all staff take responsibility for the veteran's experience and attempt to resolve complaints at the lowest level possible in the organization. To implement a proactive model, OPCC&CT recommended that this VAMC consider developing processes to increase the engagement of VAMC staff external to the patient advocacy program, such as physicians.

governance.[22] To do so, an agency may develop an organizational structure that assigns responsibilities to discrete units and defines reporting lines at all levels of the organization. Without providing specific, timely guidance to VAMCs on the governance of the patient advocacy program, the program is at risk of not meeting its minimum expectations.

In light of the limited and outdated guidance on the governance of the program, patient advocacy program staff at most of our selected VAMCs noted that the VAMC department to which patient advocates report can have a direct effect on the ability of staff to resolve veterans' complaints. For example, patient advocates at one VAMC said because of the program's position within the organization, they did not have the authority to ensure that VAMC officials external to the patient advocacy program, such as physicians, quickly engaged in responding to veterans' complaints. In these cases, a patient advocate would contact the physician to resolve a complaint, but may not have received a response until the matter was brought to the attention of the physician's supervisor—a reporting line that is outside of the patient advocacy program at this VAMC. Officials from several of our selected VAMCs and VSOs noted that the position of the patient advocacy program within VAMCs may not give patient advocates the authority to require VAMC staff to respond to veterans' complaints. They added that conflict-of-interest concerns could arise when a veteran has a complaint about a VAMC for which the patient advocate works. (See app. III for additional information on the governance of the patient advocacy program at selected VAMCs).

In VA's written comments on a draft of this chapter, which are reproduced in Appendix IV, VA stated that it issued its new directive for the patient advocacy program that had been in development as we were conducting our review.[23] While the updated directive specifies that a VAMC's lead patient advocate should report to the facility director, it does not specify the VAMC department to which other patient advocacy program staff, including patient advocates who are not designated as lead

[22] GAO-14-704G.

[23] See Department of Veterans Affairs, Veterans Health Administration, *VHA Patient Advocacy*, VHA Directive 1003.04 (Washington, D.C.: Feb. 7, 2018).

patient advocates and service-level advocates, should report. In addition, OPA's National Strategic Workgroup recently submitted recommendations to OPA on the governance of the patient advocacy program. OPA officials stated that they plan to prioritize the recommendations and elicit feedback from VISN directors on how to operationalize the recommendations. However, it is unclear whether OPA will provide additional guidance related to the governance of the program based on these recommendations, such as guidance on the VAMC department to which all types of patient advocacy program staff should report. Until actions to address the weaknesses we found are completed, guidance on the governance of the program will continue to be lacking.

VHA Has Provided Limited Guidance to VAMCs on Staffing the Patient Advocacy Program

VHA has provided limited guidance to VAMCs on the number and type of patient advocacy program staff needed to ensure that complaints from veterans are addressed in a convenient and timely manner. According to VHA's existing handbook for the program, every VAMC should have at least one patient advocate and appropriate administrative, technical, and clerical support should be provided to allow for efficient performance of the responsibilities of program staff. OPCC&CT did not provide guidance on how VAMCs should determine the appropriate number of administrative, technical, and clerical staff or type of patient advocacy program staff, such as lead patient advocates and service-level advocates. According to officials, this was because no assessment was conducted to identify what staff resources would be needed to meet the expectations of the program. In the absence of such an assessment, OPCC&CT instead relied on each VAMC to determine what resources would be needed based on the facility's size and services provided. However, VHA's handbook for the program does not provide instruction for VAMC or VISN officials on how to determine the number and type of staff needed for the program. OPCC&CT officials added that budget constraints can also affect a

VAMC's ability to hire the appropriate staff for the program. (See app. III for additional information on the number and type of patient advocacy program staff at selected VAMCs).

Officials at all but one of the selected VAMCs stated that program staff at their VAMCs had more work to do than they could handle. For example, VAMC officials cited backlogs in work, such as calls from veterans not being answered, messages not being responded to, voicemail boxes being full, and not all veterans' feedback being entered into PATS. Officials from one VAMC we spoke with in July 2017 stated that due to workload demands and not enough patient advocacy program staff at their VAMC, they had roughly 300 unanswered phone calls at that time from veterans who want to provide feedback to a patient advocate. Officials from several VSOs we spoke with stated that there is not enough patient advocate staff, adding that veterans reported that their calls to patient advocates were not answered, they were unable to reach an advocate, or their calls were not responded to in a timely manner.

The lack of staffing guidance is inconsistent with GAO's *Key Principles for Effective Strategic Workforce Planning*, which states that workforce planning is essential to addressing an organization's critical need to align its human capital program with its current and emerging mission and programmatic goals.[24] Further, federal internal control standards require agencies to design control activities to achieve objectives, a key aspect of effectively staffing a program.[25] Such control activities may include effectively managing the agency's workforce, such as by continually assessing the knowledge, skills, and abilities of the workforce to achieve organizational goals.

The lack of guidance on staffing may impede VAMCs' efforts to ensure that they have the appropriate number and type of staff to administer the patient advocacy program. The resulting misalignment of

---

[24] See GAO *Human Capital: Key Principles for Effective Strategic Workforce Planning,* GAO-04-39 (Washington, D.C.: Dec. 11, 2003). As part of the planning process, organizations should determine the skills and competencies that will be needed to achieve current and future programmatic results and develop strategies, such as policies and practices that are tailored to address the gaps in number, deployment, and alignment of human capital approaches.

[25] GAO-14-704G.

staff resources could have negatively affected VAMCs' ability to achieve the program's objectives, including addressing veterans' complaints in a timely manner. For example, if there are not a sufficient number of patient advocates to respond to veterans' phone calls in a timely manner, VAMCs may not be able to ensure that patient advocates can respond to veterans' complaints within 7 days, as called for by VHA's handbook for the program.

According to VHA officials, OPA analyzed feedback from VAMCs on the factors that should be considered in developing national guidelines for staffing, such as facility size and complexity level, and directed its National Strategic Workgroup to develop recommendations for determining the extent to which VAMCs have utilized various patient advocacy program staff, such as service-level advocates, by the spring of 2018. However, OPA expects that these efforts will result in recommendations for consideration, and it is unclear what steps, if any, will be taken based on the recommendations. Until actions to address the weaknesses we found are completed, the lack of guidance for VAMCs on determining the appropriate number and types of staff will put the patient advocacy program at risk of being unable to address veterans' complaints in a convenient and timely manner.

VHA Has Recommended Training for Patient Advocates, But Has Not Developed an Approach to Routinely Assess Their Training Needs or Monitored Training Completion

VHA Has Developed a Recommended Training List for Patient Advocates, but Has Not Developed an Approach to Assess Their Training Needs on a Routine Basis

VHA has recently developed a list of recommended training for patient advocates. In the spring of 2017, OPCC&CT officials updated a recommended training list for patient advocates developed before 2011 when OPCC&CT began overseeing the patient advocacy program. The training list covers a wide variety of topics, including how to enter and examine trends in PATS data, as well as key responsibilities of patient advocates outlined in VHA's handbook for the program. OPCC&CT officials stated that they would like to make the trainings required, but have not pursued this because of the lengthy process within VHA to designate required training for a specific group of staff. To update the list in 2017, OPCC&CT convened a workgroup (which included several patient advocates) to determine whether the old training list was sufficient, and the workgroup shared its suggested updates with VISN level coordinators for distribution to VAMCs in April 2017.

We found that OPCC&CT has not developed an approach to routinely assess the training needs of patient advocates. Rather, OPCC&CT officials stated that they relied on VAMC and VISN staff to conduct these assessments. However, VHA's handbook for the program does not specify that VAMC or VISN officials are responsible for conducting routine assessments of patient advocates' training needs. None of our selected VAMCs routinely conducted assessments of the training needs of patient advocates, such as assessing whether advocates were adequately trained to carry out their responsibilities. Officials from two VAMCs said they used ad hoc approaches to assess training needs. For example, one patient advocate supervisor stated that training is offered on an "as needed" basis in patient advocate meetings when a training need is identified.

The lack of an approach for routinely assessing the training needs of patient advocates is inconsistent with federal standards for internal control related to control activities.[26] Under these standards relating to human capital, management ensures that training is aimed at developing and retaining employee knowledge, skills, and abilities to meet changing organizational needs. Management should also continually assess the knowledge, skills, and ability needs of a program so that the program is able to obtain a workforce that has the required knowledge, skills, and abilities to achieve organizational goals.

---

[26] GAO-14-704G.

Without an approach for routinely assessing the training needs of patient advocates, VHA may not be able to clearly identify gaps in the knowledge and skills of these staff over time, which, in turn, could put the program at risk of not meeting its goals. For example, if there is a gap in understanding among patient advocates that all complaints should be entered into PATS, addressing veterans' complaints may be delayed, if addressed at all, and opportunities to analyze complaint data for the purpose of identifying system-wide improvements may be missed.

According to VHA officials, OPA analyzed feedback from VAMCs on the training needs of patient advocates, including how to correctly enter data into PATS, and directed its National Strategic Workgroup to develop recommendations for assessing the training needs of patient advocates by the spring of 2018. OPA expects that these efforts will result in recommendations for OPA to consider, but it is unclear what steps, if any, will be taken based on the recommendations. Until actions to address the weaknesses we found are completed, the lack of routine assessments of training needs will continue to put the program at risk of staff not having the requisite skills and knowledge to carry out their duties.

VHA Has Not Monitored Training Completion for Patient Advocates

VHA has not monitored the completion of training for patient advocates. Specifically, OPCC&CT officials said that they did not monitor the extent to which patient advocates completed the recommended training distributed in April 2017. Instead, these officials relied on patient advocate supervisors to monitor training completion. However, VHA's handbook for the program does not specify that patient advocate supervisors are responsible for monitoring the completion of training for patient advocates.

Half of patient advocate supervisors at our selected VAMCs did not track the completion of patient advocacy training. Patient advocate supervisors said that they are able to track the completion of general VA employee training through VA's Talent Management System. However, most training specific to patient advocacy were generally not included in this system during the period of our review. Officials from our selected VAMCs who did track patient advocacy training used various methods to record completion, such as keeping attendance lists for the training provided.

Taking steps to monitor training completion would be consistent with GAO's *Guide for Assessing Strategic Training and Development Efforts in the Federal Government* which identifies components of the training and development process, including having agencies collect and monitor data corresponding to establishing training objectives.[27] Monitoring training completion would also be consistent with federal standards for internal control related to control activities.[28] Under these standards relating to human capital, management ensures that training is aimed at developing and retaining employee knowledge, skills, and abilities to meet changing organizational needs. Management also continually assesses the knowledge, skills, and ability needs of a program so that the program is able to obtain a workforce that has the required knowledge, skills, and abilities to achieve organizational goals—key components for monitoring training completion.

If patient advocates are not properly trained in how to use PATS to document and resolve complaints, tracking the status of complaints may be more difficult, which could increase the likelihood that they are not addressed in a timely manner, if at all. Further, CARA specifies that the director of OPA should ensure that patient advocates receive training specific to patient advocacy.[29]

According to VHA officials, OPA did not obtain information on whether patient advocates completed recommended training and did not identify an approach for monitoring training completion moving forward. Without monitoring training completion, there is an increased risk that patient advocates have not received the training they need to effectively

---

[27] GAO-04-546G.
[28] GAO-14-704G.
[29] Pub. L. No. 114-198, § 924, 130 Stat. 767 (2016), codified at 38 U.S.C. § 7309A(c)(2)(C).

fulfill their responsibilities such as advocating on behalf of veterans and consistently using PATS to document and resolve complaints.

VHA HAS NOT MONITORED PATIENT ADVOCACY DATA-ENTRY PRACTICES OR REVIEWED PATIENT ADVOCACY DATA TO ASSESS PROGRAM PERFORMANCE AND IDENTIFY SYSTEM-WIDE IMPROVEMENTS

VHA Has Not Monitored Whether Complaints Were Always Entered into PATS and Issue Codes Assigned Consistently

VHA officials have not monitored PATS data-entry practices to ensure complaints were always entered into PATS and issue codes were assigned consistently to ROCs. OPCC&CT officials told us they did not monitor the data-entry practices of patient advocacy program staff to ensure that all complaints were entered into PATS, a key goal according to VHA's handbook for the program.[30] Rather, they relied on VISN and VAMC officials to ensure that program staff entered all complaints into PATS. Officials from two of the five VISNs we interviewed stated that they did not perform any audits or checks of the data entered into PATS by patient program staff at VAMCs.

We also found inconsistencies in the extent to which VAMC officials entered complaints into PATS, with complaints always entered into PATS at one of our selected VAMCs, while at other VAMCs some complaints were left unrecorded, according to officials. For example, at one VAMC, officials stated that over a third of the complaints received were not entered into PATS due to the competing workload demands of patient advocates. Similarly, at another selected VAMC, almost a quarter of the complaints received were not entered into PATS, according to patient advocates there

[30] See VHA Handbook 1003.4. The handbook states that requests for information and compliments may also be entered into PATS, as this information is useful in determining common areas of confusion that could be addressed in a proactive manner.

who explained that they primarily used a document outside of PATS to record veterans' feedback.

In addition, OPCC&CT officials told us they did not monitor whether patient advocates used a consistent practice to assign issue codes to veterans' feedback recorded into PATS. Using a consistent data-entry practice is important to ensure that PATS data can be compared across VAMCs to better enable an accurate and comprehensive understanding of veterans' issues and concerns, a goal of the patient advocacy program. OPCC&CT officials stated that they relied on VISN-level coordinators to monitor coding practices because VHA's handbook for the program states that these coordinators should develop VISN-wide consistent approaches for entering complaints into PATS. VISN-level coordinators from two selected VISNs stated that they created a standard practice for assigning issue codes within a particular VISN; however, the coding practices differed between VISNs, making national level analysis difficult.

We also found inconsistencies in how VAMC officials coded specific veterans' feedback. For example, patient advocates did not use consistent practices to code issues related to the Veterans Choice Program (Choice Program), one of the most common types of issues patient advocates told us they hear about from veterans.[31] Officials from one of our selected VAMCs said they code feedback related to the Choice Program under a specific "request for information" issue code, regardless of whether the feedback was a request for information, compliment, or complaint. In contrast, officials at another VAMC stated that they typically code feedback related to the Choice Program as a complaint related to billing. (See app. II for additional information on data-entry practices at selected VAMCs).

OPCC&CT's lack of monitoring of PATS data-entry practices is inconsistent with GAO's *Assessing the Reliability of Computer-Processed Data* which identifies the importance of consistent data-entry practices to

---

[31] The Veterans Choice Program is a program that allows eligible veterans to receive health care from a community provider when faced with long wait times, lengthy travel distances, or other challenges accessing care at a VAMC.

ensure that data are reasonably complete and accurate.[32] Further, federal standards for internal control related to information and communications require agencies to use quality information, such as relevant data from reliable sources, to achieve the agency's objectives.[33] Under internal control standards for control activities, management also is to monitor performance to achieve objectives. Without OPCC&CT monitoring data-entry practices, the patient advocacy program is at risk of not meeting its goal that all complaints are entered into PATS and there is an increased likelihood of VHA not having an accurate understanding of veterans' complaints across VAMCs.

Moving forward, in fall 2017, OPA distributed meeting minutes to all VISN and VAMC directors stating that all veterans' feedback should be consistently recorded in PATS. OPA officials also updated some of the issue codes in PATS in fall 2017 and added a code specifically for community care issues, such as issues related to the Choice Program. In addition, OPA officials stated that they plan to promote the consistent assignment of issue codes to veterans' feedback through national training, but have not specified when this training will occur or if OPA staff will monitor patient advocates' consistent assignment of issue codes or of data-entry practices generally. Until these actions are completed, however, the gaps in monitoring of PATS data-entry practices that we identified will continue to exist, putting the program at risk of incomplete or unreliable data that may not allow an accurate understanding of veterans' complaints, critical to making system-wide improvements.

VHA Has Not Systematically Reviewed PATS Data to Assess Program Performance and Identify Potential System-Wide Improvements

VHA officials have not systematically reviewed PATS data to assess program performance and identify potential system-wide improvements,

[32] GAO-09-680G.
[33] GAO-14-704G.

goals of the patient advocacy program. Specifically, OPCC&CT officials stated that they reviewed PATS data in response to inquiries, but did not conduct systematic reviews of the data over time. For example, they did not track VAMC performance on responding to complaints in a timely manner or track the most common complaints across VAMCs to identify potential opportunities for system-wide improvements.

OPCC&CT officials stated that they did not conduct systematic reviews of PATS data because VISN and VAMC officials were primarily responsible for these analyses. However, according to VHA's handbook for the patient advocacy program, VHA officials have a responsibility to examine PATS data for trends across VAMCs and identify any areas for system-wide improvement. Officials stated that it was challenging to analyze PATS information included in narrative text, such as descriptions of veterans' feedback.

Not reviewing PATS data is inconsistent with federal standards for internal control for monitoring which require agencies to establish and operate monitoring activities, such as assessing the quality of performance over time, and evaluate the results.[34] Further, not conducting systematic assessments of PATS data made it difficult for OPCC&CT to determine program performance, such as whether the program was meeting its goal that all complaints are entered into PATS and responded to within 7 days. Officials explained that VHA interprets this goal to mean that complaints are closed in PATS within 7 days. According to VA, between FY 2014 and FY 2017 there were more than 53,000 complaints per year open for greater than 7 days.[35] If OPCC&CT officials had conducted systematic reviews of PATS data, they may have been able to identify that there were a significant number of complaints open for longer than 7 days and consider what actions should be taken, such as providing additional guidance to VAMCs on how to address complaints in a timely manner.

Furthermore, without systematically reviewing PATS data across VAMCs to identify potential system-wide improvements, OPCC&CT

---

[34] GAO-14-704G.

[35] According to VA, between FY 2014 and FY 2017, the total number of reports of contact entered in PATS ranged from about 360,000 to about 414,000 per year.

officials may have been unaware of important care issues across VAMCs. For example, patient advocates from several of our selected VAMCs stated that opioid prescription issues are among the most common complaints they received from veterans. If OPCC&CT officials were to have systematically reviewed PATS data across VAMCs to determine the prevalence of these types of complaints, they could have identified the need to address them on a national level and consider system-wide policies or guidance in response.

According to VHA officials, OPA is in the process of identifying the data it needs to review on a routine basis, and directed its National Strategic Workgroup to identify program data that could be reviewed to assess program performance and identify potential system-wide improvements by the spring of 2018. However, OPA expects that these efforts will result in recommendations for OPA to consider, and it is unclear what steps, if any, will be taken based on the recommendations. Until actions to address the weaknesses we found are completed, the lack of a systematic review of PATS data will persist, putting the program at continued risk of missed opportunities for identifying and addressing weaknesses across VAMCs.

CONCLUSION

As one of the largest health care delivery systems in the nation, it is critically important for VHA to ensure that each veteran who receives health care services has easy access to an advocate who listens to that veteran's feedback and responds in a timely manner. This is especially important given concerns about veterans' ability to receive timely and quality care. However, VHA's efforts to ensure that the patient advocacy program is meeting its goals—to identify potential system-wide improvements and respond to complaints within 7 days—have fallen short. OPCC&CT did not provide sufficient oversight to the program in the four key areas of governance, staffing, training, and data-entry practices, which has left the program at risk for not meeting its goals.

VHA's newly established OPA has initiated plans to improve the patient advocacy program in these four areas; however, most of these plans center around a workgroup that will make recommendations for OPA to consider, and it is unclear what specific actions, if any, will be taken based on these recommendations. Further, documentation for several of OPA's planned efforts has not been finalized. Unless specific actions to address the weaknesses we identified are completed expeditiously, the program is at risk of not meeting its goals, including addressing veterans' complaints in a convenient and timely manner. Furthermore, without addressing the weaknesses we identified, OPA misses opportunities to review PATS data across VAMCs to identify potential system-wide issues that, if addressed, could significantly improve the experience of veterans. Such reviews are critical to ensuring that VHA is taking steps to both meet its goal in its strategic plan to provide veterans with timely and quality health care, and to address recent issues it has faced, such as veterans' ability to access care in a timely manner.

RECOMMENDATIONS FOR EXECUTIVE ACTION

We are making the following six recommendations to the VHA Undersecretary for Health:

- provide updated guidance to VAMCs on the governance of the patient advocacy program, including clear definitions of reporting lines (Recommendation 1)
- assess and provide guidance to VAMCs on appropriately staffing the patient advocacy program, including guidance on how to determine the appropriate number and type of staff (Recommendation 2)
- develop an approach to routinely assess the training needs of patient advocates. (Recommendation 3)
- monitor the completion of training for patient advocates. (Recommendation 4)

- monitor PATS data-entry practices to ensure all complaints are entered into PATS and that veterans' feedback is coded consistently. (Recommendation 5)
- systematically review PATS data to assess program performance and identify potential system-wide improvements. (Recommendation 6).

AGENCY COMMENTS AND OUR EVALUATION

We provided a draft of this chapter to VA for comment. In its written comments, which are reproduced in Appendix IV, VA concurred with our recommendations and noted that it recently issued the new directive for patient advocacy that had been in development as we were conducting our review. The directive supersedes the outdated handbook for the patient advocacy program and describes certain aspects of program governance, including certain reporting lines, roles, and responsibilities. Accordingly, VA requested that we close our first recommendation related to governance. We revised our report to reflect the issuance of the new directive. However, we do not believe the directive fully implements our recommendation. While the updated directive specifies that a VAMC's lead patient advocate should report to the facility director, it does not specify the VAMC department to which other patient advocacy program staff, including patient advocates who are not designated as lead patient advocates and service-level advocates, should report. Until VA specifies the reporting lines for these other patient advocacy program staff, our recommendation will remain open. In addition, VA stated in its written comments that OPA has efforts underway related to staffing, training, and PATS data entry and assessment and provided estimated completion dates for these efforts. We will monitor VA's efforts to address our recommendations. VA did not provide technical comments.

We are sending copies of this chapter to the appropriate congressional committees, the Secretary of Veterans Affairs, the Under Secretary for Health, and other interested parties.

Debra A. Draper
Director, Health Care

APPENDIX I: AWARENESS OF THE PATIENT ADVOCACY PROGRAM

Our eight selected Department of Veterans Affairs (VA) medical centers (VAMC) use a variety of methods to make veterans or their representatives aware of the patient advocacy program, including providing brochures on the program, displaying signage, and providing program information on the VAMC's website.[36]

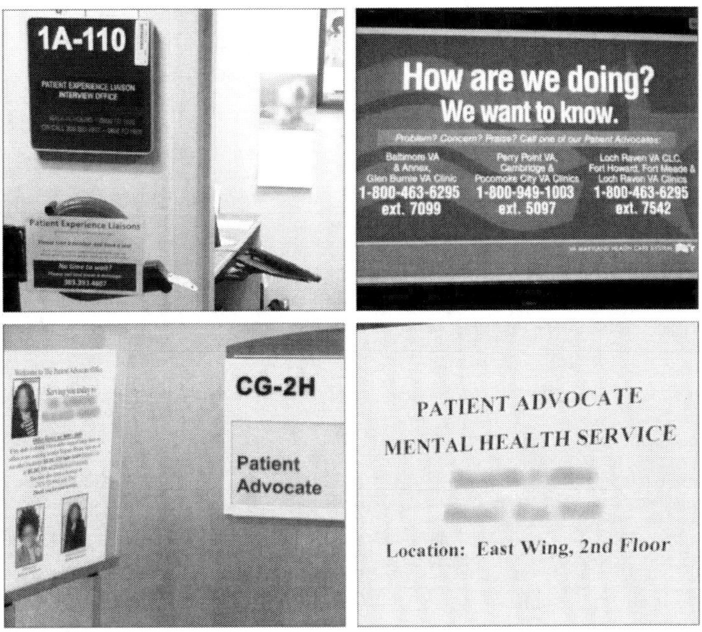

Source: GAO. | GAO-18-356.

Figure 2. Examples of Patient Advocacy Program Signage at Selected Department of Veterans Affairs Medical Centers.

[36] The term "VAMC" refers to an individual VAMC and any of its associated facilities, such as community-based outpatient clinics.

(See Figure 2 for examples of patient advocacy program signage at some of the VAMCs we visited).

APPENDIX II: PATIENT ADVOCATE TRACKING SYSTEM (PATS) DATA ENTRY AND MANAGEMENT

Patient advocacy program staff, such as patient advocates or service-level advocates who are designated to respond to veterans' feedback, enter feedback from veterans or their representatives in the Veterans Health Administration (VHA) Patient Advocate Tracking System (PATS) by creating a report of contact (ROC). Each ROC includes basic information regarding the individuals involved, a description of the feedback provided by the veteran, and a description of the steps taken to resolve the issue. Patient advocacy program staff assign one or more issue codes that generally describe the nature of the feedback, such as "coordination of care." (See Figures 3 and 4).

In order to organize veterans' feedback, VHA categorizes feedback as either requests for information, compliments, or complaints. Within each of these categories VHA defines specific issue codes for program staff to select from based on the description of the veteran's feedback. (See Table 2).

The Comprehensive Addiction and Recovery Act of 2016 (CARA), includes a provision for every VAMC to display the purpose of the program, along with the contact information of a patient advocate at the facility, in as many prominent locations as deemed appropriate to be seen by the largest percentage of veterans.[37]

In September 2016, VHA Central Office sent a memo to Veterans Integrated Service Network (VISN) directors explaining this requirement and an Office of Patient Centered Care and Cultural Transformation (OPCC&CT) official obtained confirmation from all VHA facilities that this requirement was met in October 2016.

[37] Comprehensive Addiction and Recovery Act of 2016, Pub. L. No. 114-198, § 922, 130 Stat. 695, 766-767 (2016).

Nevertheless, officials from two veterans service organizations (VSO) we interviewed stated they often encounter veterans who are not aware of the patient advocacy program.

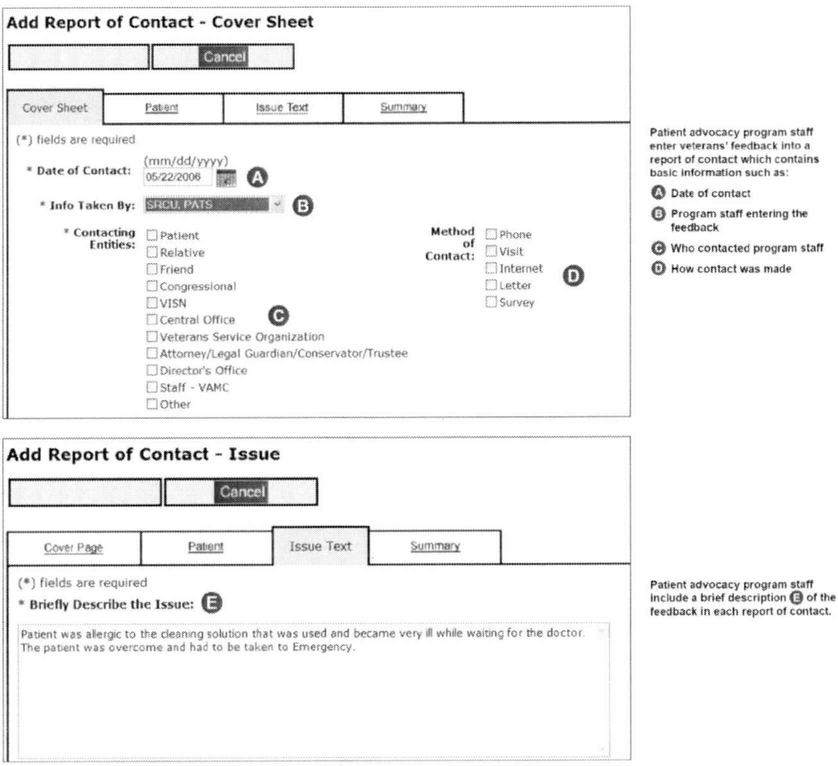

Legend: VAMC= Department of Veterans Affairs Medical Center; VISN= Veterans Integrated Service Network.

Source: GAO analysis of Veterans Health (VHA) documents and interviews with VHA officials. | GAO-18-356.

Note: In addition to contacting a patient advocate, veterans may use VA's Inquiry Routing and Information System, an Internet-based public messaging system, to express feedback.

Figure 3. Example of Information Patient Advocacy Program Staff at VAMCs Enter in the Patient Advocate Tracking System (PATS) to Add a Report of Contact (ROC).

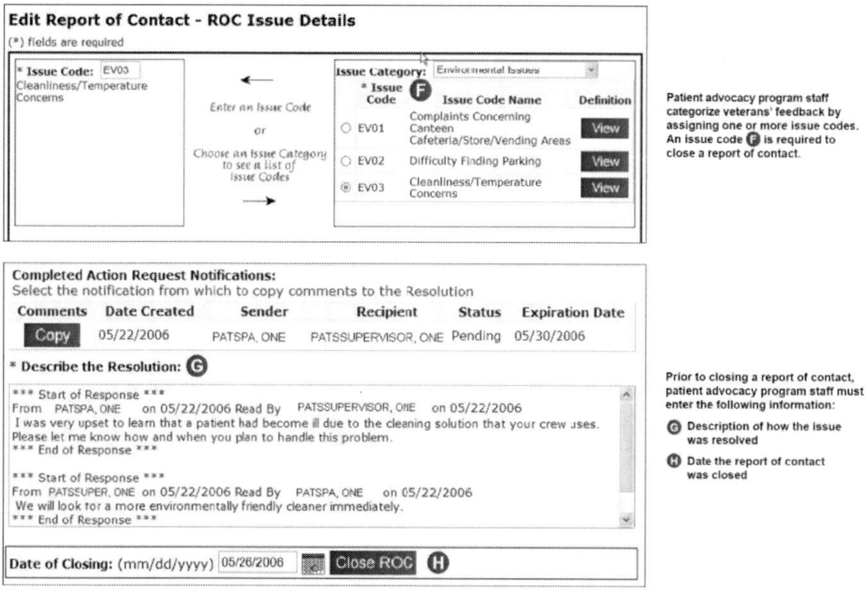

Source: GAO analysis of Veterans Health (VHA) documents and interviews with VHA officials. | GAO-18-356.

Figure 4. Example of Information Patient Advocacy Program Staff at Department of Veterans Affairs Medical Centers (VAMC) Enter in the Patient Advocate Tracking System to Close a Report of Contact (ROC).

Table 2. Issue Codes Used to Describe Veterans' Feedback in the Veterans Health Administration (VHA) Patient Advocate Tracking System (PATS), Fiscal Year (FY) 2017

Category	Issue description
Request for information	Application for care/eligibility for medical benefits
Request for information	Department of Veterans Affairs (VA) billing for service
Request for information	Advance directives
Request for information	Referral issues (internal/community)
Request for information	Medical center regulations
Request for information	Obtaining copies of medical records/completion of forms
Request for information	VA regional office questions on compensation and pension
Request for information	Legal issues
Request for information	Patient rights and responsibilities
Request for information	Other
Request for information	Social services
Compliment	Compliment received from patient/family member/staff

Category	Issue description
Complaint	Excessive wait at facility for a scheduled appointment
Complaint	Excessive wait at facility for an unscheduled appointment
Complaint	Excessive delay in scheduling or rescheduling appointment
Complaint	Delay/postponement in scheduled test/procedures or surgery
Complaint	Delay in receiving test results
Complaint	Excessive wait for care (inpatient)
Complaint	Excessive wait for equipment/wrong equipment sent
Complaint	Delay ordering/renewing pain medications
Complaint	Delay ordering/renewing other medications
Complaint	Excessive wait in pharmacy
Complaint	Excessive wait for pharmacy mailings
Complaint	Phone calls/letters/secure messages not returned/or timely
Complaint	Delay in receiving travel pay
Complaint	Delay in receiving completed forms from provider
Complaint	Appeal - denial of application
Complaint	Appeal - tier level hierarchy
Complaint	Appeal - revocation/removal from program
Complaint	All other clinical appeals (not caregiver related)
Complaint	Dissatisfied with referral outcome
Complaint	Patient perceives care is not coordinated/expectations not met
Complaint	Inconsistency in information given to patient/family
Complaint	Appointment date/time misunderstood/not communicated/wrong
Complaint	Diagnosis/care/prevention
Complaint	Purpose/side effects of medication
Complaint	Emotional needs not met
Complaint	Provider is difficult to understand
Complaint	Lack of privacy
Complaint	Complaints concerning canteen cafeteria/store/vending areas
Complaint	Difficulty finding parking
Complaint	Cleanliness/temperature/sensory concerns
Complaint	Signage not clear (directional maps etc.)
Complaint	Family not involved in patient's care
Complaint	Application for care/eligibility for medical benefits
Complaint	Eligibility for health care/follow up/hospital/extended/community living center
Complaint	Dental eligibility
Complaint	Ambulance/private hospital/private care payment eligibility
Complaint	VA billing for service/pharmacy co-payment
Complaint	Prosthetics eligibility
Complaint	Travel eligibility
Complaint	Complementary and integrative health
Complaint	Patient does not have one provider
Complaint	Patient does not know who is their provider

Table 2. (Continued)

Category	Issue description
Complaint	Hygiene, diet, feeding, therapy, ambulation needs (inpatient/health care)
Complaint	Problems with pain management
Complaint	Patient/family not included in planning care
Complaint	Patient/family disagrees about decisions on care
Complaint	Lack of confidence or trust in caregiver
Complaint	Request for non-formulary medication
Complaint	Complaints concerning medical records
Complaint	Concerns with confidentiality/privacy in medical record
Complaint	Medical center regulations
Complaint	VA regional office and/or compensation and pension issues
Complaint	Fiduciary issues
Complaint	Missing and/or damaged personal property
Complaint	Allegations of negligence/malpractice
Complaint	Allegations of abuse
Complaint	Medication error
Complaint	Issue related to safety
Category	Issue description
Complaint	Patient not treated with dignity and respect/perceived rudeness
Complaint	Perceived retaliation for expressing concerns
Complaint	Lack of coordination between inpatient and outpatient care
Complaint	Deceased patient issues by a family member
Complaint	Excessive delay of discharge/discharge too soon

Source: GAO analysis of VHA documents. | GAO-18-356.

Note: This table includes issue codes used by VHA patient advocacy program staff to document feedback recorded in PATS in fiscal year (FY) 2017. In October 2017, the Office of Patient Advocacy updated the list of issue codes in PATS for use during FY 2018. The updated list deletes some existing codes, adds new codes, and updates definitions for some existing codes.

According to VA, in fiscal year (FY) 2017, there were 268,114 veterans associated with ROCs entered in PATS.[38] VA also reported that, in the same year, patient advocacy program staff entered 414,256 unique reports of contact in PATS. According to VA, from the unique reports of contact in PATS, program staff documented 473,564 issues, which included (but were not limited to) 112,722 requests for information, 35,839

[38] VHA officials stated that veterans' feedback is not always entered in PATS, so the number of unique veterans associated with reports entered in PATS may not represent the total percentage of veterans who provide feedback to patient advocacy program staff.

compliments, and 325,003 complaints.[39] See Table 3 for the top five issues that patient advocacy program staff across VAMCs entered in PATS for FY 2017. According to VA, in FY 2017, a total of 1,391 program staff system-wide entered data in PATS. In the same year, according to PATS, veterans, rather than family members or friends, most often provided feedback to patient advocacy program staff.

Table 3. The Most Common Issues Entered in the Patient Advocate Tracking System (PATS), according to the Department of Veterans Affairs (VA), Fiscal Year 2017

Category	Issue description	Number of issues entered in PATS[a]
Request for Information	Referral issues (internal/community)	54,903
Compliment	Compliment received from patient, family member, and/or staff member	35,839
Complaint	Patient/family disagrees about decisions on care	31,718
Complaint	Phone calls/letters/secure messages not returned/answered in a timely manner	24,949
Complaint	Patient perceives care is not coordinated/expectations not met	23,617

Notes: Data presented in the table were provided by VA officials in January 2018 based on the number of issues entered in PATS in fiscal year 2017. According to Veterans Health Administration (VHA) officials involved in overseeing the patient advocacy program, patient advocates may interpret an issue description (designated by a specific issue code) differently. These differing interpretations may have contributed to the data shown in this table. In addition, VHA officials stated that veterans' feedback is not always entered in PATS, so the number of issues shown in the table may not represent all feedback that patient advocates received from veterans.

[a]Patient advocates or other VA officials can assign more than one issue code to each report of contact (ROC) entered in PATS. According to VAMC officials, multiple issue codes may be assigned to one ROC when a veteran describes multiple issues at the same time, or when there are multiple issue codes that describe a veterans' complaint. Therefore, the number of issues may not be equivalent to the number of unique ROCs for a given year.

[39] According to VA officials, these numbers are likely an underestimate of feedback provided by veterans, as not all feedback is entered in PATS.

Table 4. Patient Advocate Tracking System (PATS) Data-Entry Practices at Eight Selected Department of Veterans Affairs Medical Centers (VAMC), as of September 2017

VAMC	Number of patient advocates who entered data in PATS	Number of service-level advocates who entered data in PATS	Recorded feedback outside of PATS?	Description of issue code(s) used to record feedback related to the Veterans Choice Program[c]
A	2	0	Yes	Ambulance, private hospital, private care, payment eligibility[d]
B	6	3	Yes	—[e]
C	2	n/[a,b]	Yes	Ambulance, private hospital, private care, payment eligibility
D	1a	2	No	VA billing for service;[d] VA billing for service, pharmacy co-payment
E	4	0	Yes	—[f]
F	3	13	Yes	Dissatisfied with referral outcome
G	5	n/[a,b]	Yes	Referral issues (internal, community)[g]
H	1	10	No	—[h]

Legend: n/a = not applicable, em dash (—) = a single issue code was not identified.

Source: GAO summary of information from selected VAMCs. | GAO-18-356.

Notes: The PATS is VA's electronic system for documenting and tracking veterans' complaints and other feedback. The term "VAMC" refers to an individual VAMC and any of its associated facilities, such as community-based outpatient clinics. Service-level advocates, such as nurses or administrative staff, are designated at some VAMCs to respond to veterans' feedback before involving a patient advocate.

[a]VAMC officials stated that in addition to one patient advocate, there are six quality management staff that serve as back up to the patient advocate and enter information into PATS.

[b]This VAMC did not utilize designated service-level advocates as part of the patient advocacy program.

[c]The Veterans Choice Program is a program that allows eligible veterans to receive health care from a community provider when faced with long wait times, lengthy travel distances, or other challenges accessing care at a VAMC.

[d]In addition to using the issue codes listed, VAMC officials stated they created a special entry in the PATS facility drop-down menu to code Veterans Choice Program feedback. When officials enter a report of contact (ROC) in PATS, each VAMC has a drop-down menu of locations within their VAMC that they populate for each ROC. According to VA officials, this is one of the only categories within PATS that VAMC employees are able to change.

[e]VAMC officials stated that there was no single code or codes used to categorize Veterans Choice Program feedback, but added the Veterans Choice Program to the medical service drop-down menu within PATS.

[f]VAMC officials stated that there was no single code or codes used to categorize Veterans Choice Program feedback.

[g]This issue code is used for requests for information with no associated complaints.

[h]VAMC officials stated they created a special entry in the PATS facility drop-down menu to code Veterans Choice Program feedback.

Our eight selected VAMCs varied in the number of patient level advocates and service-level advocates who had access to PATS, whether veterans' feedback was recorded outside of PATS, and which issue code or codes were used to record feedback related to the Veterans Choice Program.[40] (See Table 4).

Examples of methods that patient advocates and service-level advocates used at selected VAMCs to record veterans' feedback outside of PATS included call logs and tracking spreadsheets. VAMC officials indicated that recording information outside of PATS helped them track their responses to veterans' feedback. Some of the information recorded outside of PATS was additional information that is not required to be entered into PATS, such as requests for information.[41]

APPENDIX III: APPROACHES TO THE GOVERNANCE AND STAFFING OF THE PATIENT ADVOCACY PROGRAM

The eight Department of Veterans Affairs (VA) medical centers (VAMC) selected for our review used a variety of approaches to govern the patient advocacy program, resulting in differences in the number of positions for patient advocates and service-level advocates and the title of the positions. Service-level advocates, such as nurses or administrative staff, are designated at some VAMCs to respond to veterans' feedback before involving a patient advocate. (See Table 5).

---

[40] The Veterans Choice Program is a program that allows eligible veterans to receive health care from a community provider when faced with long wait times, lengthy travel distances, or other challenges accessing care at a VAMC.

[41] The Veterans Choice Program is a program that allows eligible veterans to receive health care from a community provider when faced with long wait times, lengthy travel distances, or other challenges accessing care at a VAMC.

Table 5. The Number of Positions and Titles Used for Patient Advocates and Service-Level Advocates at Eight Selected Department of Veterans Affairs Medical Centers (VAMC), as of September 2017

VAMC	Patient advocates		Service-level advocates	
	Number of positions	Title	Number of positions	Title
A	2	Patient advocate	28	Service-level liaison
B	6	Patient experience liaison	29	Service-level advocate
C	2	Patient representative	0	Service line champion
D	1	Patient representative	16	Patient advocate liaison
E	4a	Patient advocate	57	Patient advocate liaison
F	3	Patient representative	86	Service-level advocate
G	9b	Patient advocate	0	Service-level advocate
H	1	Patient representative	10	Service line patient experience liaison

Source: GAO summary of information from selected VAMCs. | GAO-18-356.

Notes: The term "VAMC" refers to an individual VAMC and any of its associated facilities such as community-based outpatient clinics. Service-level advocates, such as nurses or administrative staff, are designated at some VAMCs to respond to veterans' feedback before involving a patient advocate.

[a]This VAMC also has four patient advocates who only handle complaints related to non-VA care. Since these patient advocates report outside of the VAMC's patient advocacy program, we did not include them in the count of patient advocates. According to an official from this VAMC, these advocates do not enter veterans' feedback in PATS.

[b]This VAMC also has two assistant patient advocates who help the patient advocates respond to veterans' feedback. These assistants are not included in the number of patient advocates.

Patient advocates reported to a variety of departments among our selected VAMCs. At two of the VAMCs, patient advocates reported to the customer or consumer relations department, while at three, patient advocates reported to the quality management department. In addition, the placement of the department that patient advocates reported to within the VAMC differed. For example, the patient advocate supervisor at one of the selected VAMCs said that patient advocates reported to the customer service manager, who did not report directly to the VAMC director. At another VAMC, the patient advocate reported directly to the VAMC director. In addition to the Veterans Health Administration (VHA) handbook for the patient advocacy program, all eight of our selected

VAMCs developed their own policies for the administration of the program, and these policies varied. For example, while almost all of the policies specified the responsibilities with respect to the patient advocacy program of the service chiefs—officials who oversee the administration and operation of service lines such as primary care, these responsibilities varied. For example, two of the policies required service chiefs to incorporate veterans' feedback into performance measures used for VAMC staff external to the patient advocacy program, such as physicians, while the other policies did not.

We also found variation between our selected VAMCs with respect to whether they had written descriptions of the service-level advocates' roles. Of the six VAMCs that designated service-level advocates, three had written descriptions of their roles, while three did not. Further, among the VAMCs that had a written description of the role of a service-level advocate, the expectations for these advocates varied. For example, one VAMC's written description specified that service-level advocates are expected to enter veterans' feedback into PATS within 7 days of receiving the feedback. The written descriptions at the other two VAMCs did not specify this expectation.

APPENDIX IV: COMMENTS FROM THE DEPARTMENT OF VETERANS AFFAIRS

DEPARTMENT OF VETERANS AFFAIRS
WASHINGTON DC 20420

March 20, 2018

Ms. Debra Draper
Director
Health Care
U.S. Government Accountability Office
441 G Street, NW
Washington, DC 20548

Dear Ms. Draper:

The Department of Veterans Affairs (VA) has reviewed the Government Accountability Office's (GAO) draft report, ***"VA HEALTH CARE: Improved Guidance and Oversight Needed for the Patient Advocacy Program"*** (GAO-18-356).

The enclosure sets forth the actions to be taken to address the GAO draft report recommendations.

VA appreciates the opportunity to comment on your draft report.

Sincerely,

Jacquelyn Hayes-Byrd
Deputy Chief of Staff

Department of Veterans Affairs (VA) Comments to
Government Accountability Office (GAO) Draft Report
"VA HEALTH CARE: Improved Guidance and Oversight Needed for the Patient Advocacy Program"
(GAO-18-356)

Recommendation 1: Provide updated guidance to VAMCs on the governance of the patient advocacy program, including clear definitions of reporting lines.

VA Comment: Concur. On February 7, 2018, the Veterans Health Administration (VHA) provided updated guidance to the Veterans Affairs (VA) medical centers with the signing of VHA Directive 1003.4, *VHA Patient Advocacy* (Attachment A). The Directive identifies governance of the patient advocacy program, including reporting lines, roles, and responsibilities. VHA considers this recommendation fully implemented and requests closure.

Recommendation 2: Assess and provide guidance to VAMCs on appropriately staffing the patient advocacy program, including guidance on how to determine the appropriate number and type of staff.

VA Comment: Concur. Staffing guidelines and ratios are being developed. The Office of Patient Advocacy (OPA) national strategic workgroup is developing recommendations on staffing ratios based on industry benchmarks, facility complexity, total number of unique Veterans served and other key factors. These recommendations will be utilized to develop initial guidelines and be incorporated into a more detailed assessment to validate and refine the staffing model. The status is in process with a target completion date of May 2018.

Recommendation 3: Develop an approach to routinely assess the training needs of patient advocates.

VA Comment: Concur. OPA is developing a process for routinely assessing the training needs of patient advocates. The first phase of the process includes collecting input from the Veterans Integrated Service Network (VISN)-level coordinators and facility patient advocates (the initial baseline assessment was done in September 2017). The next step involves quarterly solicitation of input from VISN-level coordinators and patient advocates on monthly community of practice calls. OPA's national strategic workgroup is developing guidelines on core competencies and a training program model. These recommendations will be used to develop formal policies and guidelines to ensure continuous assessment of training needs and validation of training effectiveness. The status is in process with a target completion date of September 2018.

Recommendation 4: Monitor the completion of training for patient advocates.

VA Comment: Concur. OPA has implemented a systematic process to monitor the completion of national trainings. Within the Talent Management System, patient advocacy training documents the name of the employee, title and date/time of training completion. For face-to-face trainings, attendees must sign a daily attendance sheet for documentation of completion.

In the VHA Directive on Patient Advocacy, supervisors/managers for patient advocates are responsible for ensuring local training of patient advocates is monitored and documented.

OPA is currently developing processes and guidelines for training compliance documentation and monitoring. The status is in process with a target completion date of September 2018.

Recommendation 5: Monitor PATS data entry practices to ensure all complaints are entered into PATS and that veterans' feedback is coded consistently.

VA Comment: Concur. Although progress has been made, monitoring of the Patient Advocate Tracking System (PATS) data entry practices continues to be developed. New issue codes and definitions were deployed on October 1, 2017, based on feedback and input from patient advocates, VISN-level coordinators and other key program stakeholders. OPA performs a quarterly review of PATS data for systemic documentation compliance and accuracy issues that need follow-up, clarification or resolution. Further monitoring of PATS data entry and coding practices is being explored and developed. The status is in process with a target completion date of July 2018.

Recommendation 6: Systematically review PATS data to assess program performance and identify potential system-wide improvements.

VA Comment: Concur. OPA has already started a systematic review of PATS data with the analysis of the first quarter, fiscal year (FY) 2018 data. With the revision and deployment of issue codes and definitions on October 1, 2017, OPA will be able to better trend issues and identify potential system-wide improvements, as further quarterly reports are reviewed and analyzed.

An OPA national strategic workgroup was chartered in September 2017 to develop recommendations on key performance indicators to help shape a framework for continuous improvement that includes identifying strong practices for dissemination, issues and opportunities, and actions to drive change. All recommendations have been received, and OPA is incorporating the recommendations into its FY 2018/FY 2019 action plan. The status is in process with a target completion date of November 2018 for implementation of actions.

In: Improvements Needed in the VA … ISBN: 978-1-53615-971-4
Editor: Charles Copeland

Chapter 8

VA HEALTH CARE: ACTIONS NEEDED TO IMPROVE OVERSIGHT OF COMMUNITY-BASED OUTPATIENT CLINICS*

United States Government Accountability Office

ABBREVIATIONS

CBOC	community-based outpatient clinic
HEDIS	Healthcare Effectiveness Data and Information Set
VA	Department of Veterans Affairs
VAMC	VA medical center
VAST	VHA site tracking
VHA	Veterans Health Administration
VISN	Veterans Integrated Service Network

* This is an edited, reformatted and augmented version of United States Government Accountability Office, Report to Congressional Requesters, Publication No. GAO-18-375, dated April 2018.

WHY GAO DID THIS STUDY

In fiscal year 2016, VHA's 733 CBOCs provided care to more than 3 million veterans at a cost of $5.3 billion. Although most of these clinics are VHA-owned and -operated, 101 are operated through contracts with non-VHA organizations. VHA policy states that CBOCs, whether VHA-operated or contracted, must provide one standard of care that is of high quality.

GAO was asked to review VHA's use of contracts to carry out core functions. This chapter examines, among other issues, the extent to which VHA oversees CBOC operations.

To conduct this work, GAO reviewed VHA's policies and CBOC Report. GAO also interviewed officials from VHA's central office and from a nongeneralizable sample of eight CBOCs and their four respective VAMCs and VISNs. The CBOCs were selected for variation in factors such as contract status and geographic area.

WHAT GAO RECOMMENDS

GAO recommends that VHA (1) implement oversight requirements that align with existing policy; (2) establish a process to ensure the CBOC Report is accurate and complete; (3) provide guidance or training to VISNs and VAMCs on how to use the CBOC Report; and (4) require use of the CBOC Report as an oversight tool. VA concurred with all of GAO's recommendations and identified actions it is taking to implement them.

WHAT GAO FOUND

Community-based outpatient clinics (CBOC) are an important part of the Department of Veterans Affairs' (VA) Veterans Health Administration (VHA) health care delivery system. These clinics are geographically separate from VA medical centers (VAMC) and provide outpatient services, including primary care and mental health care. GAO found weaknesses in VHA's oversight of CBOCs:

- Incomplete policy implementation. VHA has not implemented certain CBOC oversight requirements as outlined in its policy. Specifically, VHA has not developed guidelines for monitoring the quality and comprehensiveness of care in CBOCs and officials said they have no plans to do so. Officials told GAO they believe the requirement was met as part of their regular oversight of Veterans Integrated Service Networks (VISN)—regional networks responsible for oversight of VAMCs and CBOCs. However, VHA may miss CBOC performance problems that are not identifiable in VISN-level data. Further, although policy requires VHA central office officials to review CBOC performance as part of quarterly VISN performance reviews, officials said they do not specifically do so unless the VISN identifies a problem. Officials from three of the four VISNs in GAO's review said they largely delegate CBOC oversight to VAMCs, and do not separately review clinic performance unless a VAMC identifies a problem.
- An inaccurate and incomplete CBOC Report. VHA's CBOC Report is prepared by VHA central office and distributed to VISNs and VAMCs quarterly and at year-end. The CBOC Report could be useful to compare clinical quality of care between VHA-operated and contracted CBOCs, but it is inaccurate and incomplete. Specifically, VHA officials have used their judgment to classify certain sites as CBOCs in the report, rather than use the official classifications in policy. GAO found that 22 percent of sites were incorrectly classified as CBOCs when they were other types of sites, including VAMCs. As a result, the report is of limited usefulness to VHA as an oversight tool.
- Lack of guidance or training on the CBOC Report. VHA central office officials do not provide guidance or training specific to understanding the CBOC Report to assist VISNs and VAMCs in their oversight of CBOCs. GAO found that in several places in the

report, shorthand text and acronyms were used, but not defined. In addition, several VISN and VAMC officials stated that guidance or training would be helpful.

- No requirement to use the CBOC Report. VHA officials told GAO that VAMCs and VISNs are expected to use the CBOC Report as an oversight tool, but GAO found that VHA lacks a requirement that they do so. Officials from three of the four VISNs and three of the four VAMCs in GAO's review were not using the report.

These weaknesses potentially lead to inconsistent oversight and create a risk that VHA is not providing one standard of care that is of high quality to veterans across VHA-operated and contracted CBOCs.

April 12, 2018
Congressional Requesters

The Department of Veterans Affairs' (VA) Veterans Health Administration (VHA) operates one of the largest health care delivery systems in the United States. In fiscal year 2016, VHA's health care system included 168 VA medical centers (VAMC) that offered inpatient, outpatient, and residential services and 733 community-based outpatient clinics (CBOC)—stand-alone clinics that are geographically separate from VAMCs and provide outpatient primary care, mental health care, and, in some cases, specialty care services. In fiscal year 2016, these clinics provided care to more than 3 million veterans at a cost of $5.3 billion, which represented about half of the veterans treated by VHA and nearly 10 percent of total spending for their care. Although most CBOCs (632 of the 733) are owned and operated by VHA, about 14 percent (101) are operated by non-VHA health care organizations that contract with VHA to provide services.[1] According to VHA, as of the end of fiscal year 2016, 29

[1] The Veterans' Health Care Eligibility Reform Act of 1996 authorizes the Department of Veterans Affairs to obtain health care resources by entering into contracts or other agreements with any health care facility, entity, or individual. Pub. L. No. 104-262, § 301, 110 Stat. 3177, 3191 (1996). Veterans Health Administration policy for acquisition of health care resources through contracting is documented in Department of Veterans Affairs,

contractors held CBOC contracts, for which VHA spent nearly $312 million.[2] It is VHA policy that all CBOCs provide one standard of care that is of high quality, regardless of whether they are VHA-operated or contracted.

In May 2000, VHA published the last in a series of reports in response to a 1998 request from the Under Secretary for Health to evaluate CBOC performance.[3] The evaluation found that VHA-operated and contracted CBOCs performed equally on most performance measures, but contracted clinics provided fewer primary care visits, had fewer patients with mental health diagnoses, and did not have adequate cost data available to compare their costs to those clinics operated by VHA. Since that time, outpatient care use in VHA has grown substantially. In 2015, an external assessment of VHA reported that between 2007 and 2014, VHA outpatient visits increased 41 percent while inpatient bed days declined 9 percent.[4] The 2015 assessment also reported that VHA's planning models predicted inpatient bed days would decline by at least another 50 percent over the next 20 years.

We and others have cited longstanding concerns about VHA's oversight of its health care system. These concerns contributed to veterans' health care being placed on GAO's High-Risk List beginning in 2015.[5]

Health Care Resources Contracting – Buying, VHA Directive 1663. (Washington, D.C.: Aug. 10, 2006).

[2] A single contract can include multiple CBOCs and a single contractor can hold more than one CBOC contract.

[3] A. Hedeen et al., *CBOC Performance Evaluation, Performance Report 3: Quality of Care Measures Based on Medical Review,* a report prepared for the Department of Veterans Affairs, May 2000.

[4] McKinsey & Company Inc., *Independent Assessment of the Health Care Delivery Systems and Management Processes of the Department of Veterans Affairs, Assessment K (Facilities),* (Sept.1, 2015). The assessment was mandated by the Veterans Access, Choice, and Accountability Act of 2014. Pub. L. No. 113-146, § 201(a)(1), 128 Stat. 1754, 1769-71 (2014). It included 12 specific assessment areas and, according to VA, resulted in 188 recommendations for reforming VHA. See Centers for Medicare & Medicaid Services Alliance to Modernize Healthcare Federally Funded Research and Development Center, *Independent Assessment of the Health Care Delivery Systems and Management Processes of the Department of Veterans Affairs, Volume I: Integrated Report* (Sept. 1, 2015).

[5] GAO maintains a high-risk list to focus attention on government agencies and programs that it identifies as high risk due to their greater vulnerabilities to fraud, waste, abuse, and mismanagement or the need for transformation to address economy, efficiency, or effectiveness challenges. GAO, *High-Risk Series: Progress on Many High-Risk Areas,*

You asked us to conduct a management review of VHA that included, among other issues, its use of contracts to carry out core functions.[6] In this chapter, we examine the extent to which:

1. VHA-operated and contracted CBOCs vary in their provision of health care services; and
2. VHA oversees CBOC operations, including ensuring the same quality of care at both VHA-operated and contracted CBOCs.

To determine the extent to which VHA-operated and contracted CBOCs vary in their provision of health care services, we analyzed fiscal years 2014 through 2016 expenditure and encounter data (the three most recent fiscal years of data available) for the 687 of 733 CBOCs that provided care as of September 30, 2016, and for which these data were available.[7] We compared expenditures per encounter and the types of

---

While Substantial Effort Needed on Others, GAO-17-317 (Washington, D.C.: Feb. 15, 2017).

[6] We have previously issued several reports that addressed specific aspects of VHA's management, including those pertaining to its policy management, human capital management, strategic planning, and organizational structure. See GAO, *Veterans Health Care: Additional Actions Could Further Improve Policy Management,* GAO-17-748 (Washington, D.C.: Sept. 22, 2017); *Veterans Affairs: Improved Management Processes Are Necessary for IT Systems That Better Support Health Care*, GAO-17-384 (Washington, D.C.: June 21, 2017); *VA Health Care: Improvements Needed in Data and Monitoring of Clinical Productivity and Efficiency*, GAO-17-480 (Washington, D.C.: May 24, 2017); *Veterans Health Administration: Management Attention Is Needed to Address Systemic, Long-standing Human Capital Challenges*, GAO-17-30 (Washington D.C.: Dec. 23, 2016); *Veterans Health Care: Improvements Needed in Operationalizing Strategic Goals and Objectives*, GAO-17-50 (Washington D.C.: Oct. 21, 2016); and *VA Health Care: Processes to Evaluate, Implement, and Monitor Organizational Structure Changes Needed*, GAO-16-803 (Washington D.C.: Sept. 27, 2016).

[7] VHA requires all facilities to record and report data on expenditures and encounters in VHA's managerial cost accounting system. VHA defines an encounter as a professional contact between a patient and a practitioner vested with responsibility for diagnosing, evaluating, and treating the patient's condition. Encounters can occur in both the outpatient and inpatient settings, and can include face-to-face interactions or those accomplished through telecommunications technology. Of 733 CBOCs providing care as of September 30, 2016, we analyzed encounter and expenditure data from 687 CBOCs—589 that were VHA-operated and 98 that were contracted. Data were not available for 46 CBOCs because, according to VHA officials, encounter and expenditure data for these CBOCs were combined with data from the VAMC and could not be reliably separated. Further, 24 of the 687 CBOCs included in our analysis did not have 3 full fiscal years of data because they

services provided by VHA-operated clinics to those for contracted clinics.[8] We also spoke to officials from VHA's central office about the factors that influence per-encounter expenditure variation across CBOCs. Given that our 3-year analysis period was relatively short, we did not adjust the values for inflation. We assessed the reliability of the encounter and expenditure data by checking for missing values and obvious errors and discussing them with VHA officials who were knowledgeable about the data. We analyzed the data as reported by CBOCs in VHA's managerial cost accounting system and we did not independently verify the accuracy or completeness of the information, or the methodology used by VHA to calculate total costs for VHA-operated clinics.[9] After taking these steps, we determined the data were sufficiently reliable for the purposes of this reporting objective.

In addition, we interviewed officials from eight selected CBOCs and from the four VAMCs and the four Veterans Integrated Service Networks (VISN) that oversee them.[10] We also interviewed the four VHA contracting officers associated with the contracted CBOCs.[11] The eight selected clinics are a nongeneralizable sample of four pairs of VHA-operated and contracted CBOCs. (See Table 1.) We selected these clinics from a list of CBOCs that

---

were new sites that began operating during the time period; we included data that were available.

[8] VHA pays contracted CBOCs a capitated per-member per-month rate that combines both direct and indirect expenditures—that is, a rate that covers the contractors' direct expenditures of providing care, as well as other indirect expenditures, such as overhead. These direct and indirect expenditures for contracted CBOCs cannot be separated from one another in VHA's managerial cost accounting system, unlike for VHA-operated CBOCs. Therefore, we examined total expenditures, which include both direct and indirect expenditures. For the VHA-operated CBOCs, we did not evaluate the methodology used by VHA to allocate indirect expenditures.

[9] GAO has previously found that challenges exist in accurately determining the costs performed by federal versus contractor personnel. See GAO, *Human Capital: Opportunities Exist to Further Improve DOD's Methodology for Estimating the Costs of Its Workforces*, GAO-13-792 (Washington, D.C.: Sept. 25, 2013).

[10] VHA organizes its system of care into regional networks called VISNs. Each VISN is responsible for coordination and oversight of all administrative and clinical activities within its specified geographic region. Specifically, the 18 VISNs oversee the day-to-day functions of VAMCs and CBOCs within their geographical regions.

[11] Each contracted CBOC is assigned a VHA contracting officer who works with the VISN and the VAMC to oversee the contract. We also spoke to two of the three contractors that administered the contracted CBOCs in our review; the third contractor was not available to speak with us during the time frame of our review.

provided services as of March 10, 2017—the most recently available data at the time of our review—using data from the VHA site tracking (VAST) system, which lists all facilities and their characteristics. We selected the clinics for variation in geographic diversity, parent VAMC complexity level, clinic type (multi-specialty vs. primary care), and clinic size.[12] We also interviewed officials from the American Legion, a veterans service organization, to obtain the perspective of veterans on the services provided at CBOCs. The information from our interviews is not generalizable to all CBOCs, VAMCs, VISNs, or contracting officers. We assessed the reliability of the VAST system data on clinic characteristics by reviewing relevant documentation and speaking to knowledgeable agency officials. We also performed data reliability checks, such as examining the data for missing values and obvious errors to test the internal consistency and reliability of the data. After taking these steps, we determined the data were reliable for the purposes of selecting sites and determining the complete list of CBOCs.

To evaluate the extent to which VHA oversees CBOC operations, including ensuring the same quality of care at both VHA-operated and contracted CBOCs, we reviewed VHA policies, including Directive 1229 that establishes VHA and VISN oversight responsibilities for outpatient sites of care, including CBOCs.[13] We also reviewed and interviewed officials about VHA's CBOC Report that documents clinical quality of care measures for both VHA-operated and contracted clinics.[14] In addition, we analyzed the report from the first quarter of 2017—the most recently

---

[12] Both multi-specialty and primary care CBOCs provide primary care and mental health care services. Multi-specialty CBOCs provide two or more specialty care services on-site. We used the total number of encounters in fiscal year 2016 as a proxy for clinic size. VHA assigns each VAMC to one of five complexity groups (1a, 1b, 1c, 2, or 3) using a facility complexity model where level 1a facilities are the most complex and level 3 facilities are the least complex. VHA uses multiple variables to measure facility complexity in four categories: patient population served, clinical services offered, education and research complexity, and administrative complexity.

[13] Department of Veterans Affairs, Veterans Health Administration, *Planning and Operating Outpatient Sites of Care*, VHA Directive 1229. (Washington, D.C.: July 7, 2017).

[14] The CBOC Report is prepared and distributed by VHA's Reporting, Analytics, Performance, Improvements and Development office within the office of the Deputy Under Secretary for Health for Organizational Excellence. An official from this office told us that they began producing the report in 2009 to compare quality of care between VHA operated and contracted CBOCs.

available report at the time of our review—and compared CBOCs in the report against sites in the VAST system as of January 3, 2017. We also interviewed officials from VHA central office and our selected clinics (including the contracting officers for our selected contracted clinics), as well as officials from the selected clinics' VAMCs and VISNs. We assessed the oversight activities performed by VHA's central office and the VISNs in the context of the federal standards for internal control.[15]

Table 1. Site Selection for Interviews with Community-Based Outpatient Clinics (CBOC)

CBOC	State	Department of Veterans Affairs medical center (VAMC)	Veterans Integrated Service Network	Veterans Health Administration (VHA)-operated or contracted
Binghamton	NY	Syracuse VAMC	2	VHA-operated
Watertown	NY	Contracted		
Anderson	SC	William Jennings Bryan Dorn VAMC	7	VHA-operated
Rock Hill	SC	Contracted		
Gillette	WY	Sheridan VAMC	19	VHA-operated
Powell	WY	Contracted		
Fergus Falls	MN	Fargo VAMC	23	VHA-operated
Williston	ND	Contracted		

Source: GAO analysis of VHA data. | GAO-18-375.

We conducted this performance audit from February 2017 to April 2018 in accordance with generally accepted government auditing standards. Those standards require that we plan and perform the audit to obtain sufficient, appropriate evidence to provide a reasonable basis for our findings and conclusions based on our audit objectives. We believe that the evidence obtained provides a reasonable basis for our findings and conclusions based on our audit objectives.

[15] GAO, *Standards for Internal Control in the Federal Government.* GAO-14-704G (Washington, D.C.: Sept. 10, 2014). Internal control is a process effected by an entity's oversight body, management, and other personnel that provides reasonable assurance that the objectives of an entity will be achieved.

BACKGROUND

Over the last decade, VHA has increasingly provided care on an outpatient basis, including primary care and mental health care services. VHA Handbook 1006.02, *VHA Site Classifications and Definitions*, defines classifications for outpatient sites of care including CBOCs.[16] VHA's Directive 1229, *Planning and Operating Outpatient Sites of Care*, outlines the process for establishing new CBOCs.[17]

VHA's Outpatient Sites of Care

VHA provides outpatient care through CBOCs, health care centers, and other outpatient services sites, which are defined in VHA's site classification policy:[18]

- CBOCs are clinics that provide primary care and mental health care services, and also may provide specialty care services such as cardiology or neurology, in an outpatient setting. CBOCs can provide a wide array of services, ranging from a small, mainly telehealth clinic with one technician and a nurse, to a large clinic with several specialty care services and providers.[19] Each clinic is overseen by, and separate from, its VAMC; each VAMC in turn is overseen by one of 18 VISNs.

---

[16] Department of Veterans Affairs, Veterans Health Administration, *VHA Site Classifications and Definitions,* VHA Handbook 1006.02 (Washington, D.C.: Dec. 30, 2013). Classifications are tracked in VAST.

[17] VHA Directive 1229.

[18] VHA Handbook 1006.02.

[19] Telehealth refers to clinical services provided remotely via telecommunications technologies. For more information on how telehealth is used in VA and other federal programs, see GAO, *Health Care: Telehealth and Remote Patient Monitoring Use in Medicare and Selected Federal Programs,* GAO-17-365 (Washington, D.C.: Apr. 14, 2017).

- Health care centers are large multi-specialty outpatient clinics that provide primary care, mental health care, and on-site surgical services, in addition to other health care services.
- Other outpatient services sites provide nonclinical services, such as social services, homelessness services, and support services. They may also provide services that are clinical in nature through telehealth or other arrangements. (See Figure 1.)

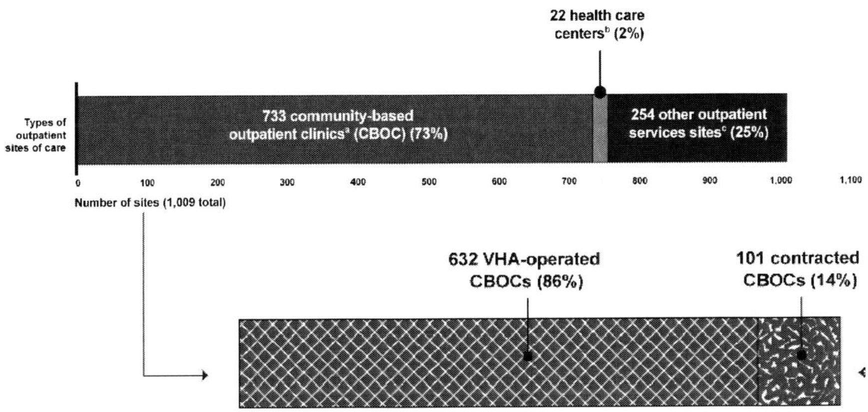

Source: GAO analysis of VHA data. | GAO-18-375.

Note: Fiscal year 2016 was the most recent complete fiscal year of data available at the time of our review.

[a]CBOCs are clinics that provide primary care and mental health care services, and also may provide specialty care services such as cardiology or neurology, in an outpatient setting.

[b]Health care centers are large multi-specialty outpatient clinics that provide primary care, mental health care, and on-site surgical services, in addition to other health care services.

[c]Other outpatient services sites provide nonclinical services, such as social services, homelessness services, and support services. They may also provide services that are clinical in nature through remote telecommunications technologies or other arrangements.

Figure 1. Veterans Health Administration (VHA) Outpatient Sites of Care, as of September 30, 2016.

VHA's Process for Establishing New CBOCs

To establish a new CBOC, VHA's policy states that the VAMC and VISN must ensure that one is needed by first exhausting existing VHA resources (such as changing clinic hours or staffing) and determining that VHA community care programs cannot meet the identified demand.[20] The VAMC and VISN follow several steps to assess the need for a new clinic:

- Step 1—The VAMC and VISN identify an underserved area using VHA models that project changes in the veteran population and trends in veterans' health care needs.
- Step 2—The VAMC develops a detailed proposal for the new clinic— an Access Expansion Plan—that includes information such as whether the proposed clinic will be VHA-operated or contracted, projected workload, scope of the services to be provided, and cost. It also describes, as required by VHA policy, how the VAMC has exhausted existing VHA resources before proposing a new clinic.
- Step 3—The VISN reviews the expansion plan, and if approved forwards it to an interdisciplinary panel at VHA's central office, which reviews it. A list of approved clinics is then sent to the Under Secretary for Health for endorsement.
- Step 4—Endorsed clinics are included in the VISN's Strategic Capital Investment Planning process submission for the fiscal year.[21] Final approval and funding for a new CBOC is dependent on Office of Management and Budget approval of VA's budget submission and VHA's final appropriations.

---

[20] VHA Directive 1229. When care is not readily accessible from VA providers, VA may purchase care from non-VA providers under various community care programs. Such care is provided under the following statutory authorities: 38 U.S.C. §§ 1703, 1725, 1728, 8111, and 8153.

[21] The Strategic Capital Investment Planning process is VHA's mechanism for planning and prioritizing capital projects. For more information on the process, see GAO, *VA Real Property: VA Should Improve Its Efforts to Align Facilities with Veterans' Needs*, GAO-17-349 (Washington, D.C.: Apr. 5, 2017).

In fiscal year 2015, VHA suspended the establishment of new CBOCs beginning in fiscal year 2018 due to several factors, including budget constraints and an emphasis on the use of VHA community care programs. However, VISNs can submit requests for exceptions to the Deputy Under Secretary for Health for Operations and Management for review. VHA officials told us 11 exceptions had been granted as of February 2018.

VHA-Operated CBOCs Provided Proportionally More Specialty Care and Had Higher Expenditures than Contracted CBOCs in Fiscal Years 2014 through 2016

VHA-Operated CBOCs Provided Proportionally More Specialty Care and Less Primary Care and Mental Health Care Than Contracted CBOCs

We found that VHA-operated CBOCs provided more specialty care and less primary care and mental health care as a proportion of their total provided services than contracted CBOCs in fiscal years 2014 through 2016. For example, in fiscal year 2016, specialty care (e.g., cardiology, gastroenterology, physical therapy) comprised 13 percent of services provided at VHA-operated clinics and 5 percent of services provided at contracted clinics. In contrast, VHA-operated clinics provided proportionally less primary care and mental health services (services offered at all CBOCs) in fiscal year 2016—these services comprised 66 percent of the services provided at VHA-operated clinics, but 84 percent of the services provided at contracted clinics. (See Figure 2.)

We found that VHA-operated CBOCs provided several specialty care services that were not offered in contracted CBOCs.

For example, dental care services and gastrointestinal endoscopy were provided by multiple VHA-operated clinics, but were not provided by any of the contracted clinics in fiscal year 2016. In addition, we found that VHA-operated clinics were generally larger and provided more complex services than contracted clinics. For example, multi-specialty CBOCs (clinics that provide two or more on-site specialty care services, and which may offer procedures requiring local anesthesia or sedation) were more often VHA operated than contracted. Of the 733 CBOCs in fiscal year 2016, 210 were classified by VHA as multi-specialty, and nearly all of these (206) were VHA-operated.

Officials from the four VAMCs and VISNs in our review told us decisions about what types of services CBOCs provide are made on a case-by-case basis according to local needs.[22] For example, officials from one VAMC told us they decided to add physical therapy specialty care to one of their VHA-operated clinics based on analysis indicating that veterans' need for this care in their community would increase. Also, officials said they wanted to alleviate the travel burden for veterans who needed the care, as the next closest VHA facility that offered this care was a 2.5-hour drive away. Officials from another VAMC told us that they approached the service needs at their clinics from a regional perspective, allowing for veteran demand for services to be met across multiple clinics in the same geographic area instead of relying on one clinic to meet the need. As a result of this approach, VAMC officials were in the process of expanding services at two of its clinics.

From fiscal years 2014 through 2016, we found that VHA-operated CBOCs had higher per-encounter expenditures than contracted CBOCs—a difference ranging from 3 to 5 percent per encounter. (See Table 2.)

---

[22] VHA policy outlines the review and approval of the expansion, reduction, or elimination of major clinical services or programs in VHA facilities including CBOCs. See Department of Veterans Affairs, Veterans Health Administration, *Restructuring of VHA Clinical Programs*, VHA Directive 1043 (Washington, D.C.: Nov. 2, 2016).

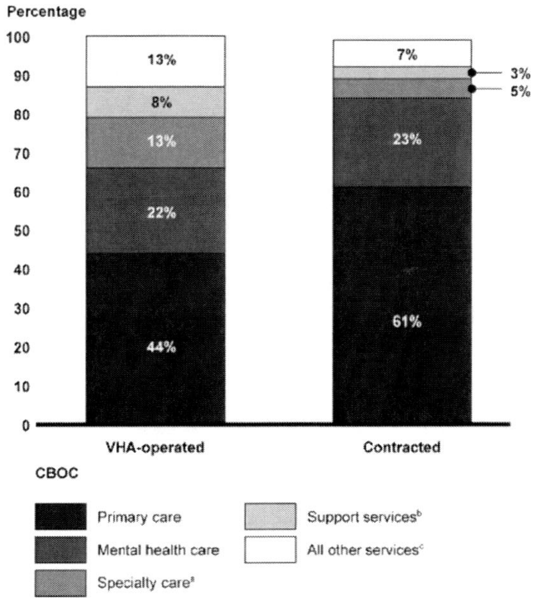

Source: GAO analysis of VHA data. | GAO-18-375.

Notes: As of September 30, 2016, there were 733 CBOCs—632 VHA-operated and 101 contracted. For these analyses, data were missing for 46 CBOCs; VHA only recorded data for these clinics at the Department of Veterans Affairs medical center level. Therefore, we analyzed data for 687 CBOCs— 589 VHA-operated and 98 contracted.

We measured services provided through encounters, which VHA defines as a professional contact between a patient and a practitioner vested with responsibility for diagnosing, evaluating, and treating the patient's condition. Encounters can occur in both the outpatient and inpatient settings, and can include face-to-face interactions or those accomplished through telecommunications technology.

Percentages do not add to 100 due to rounding.

[a]Specialty care services include cardiology, gastroenterology, and rehabilitation services (e.g., physical therapy).

[b]Support services include radiology and laboratory services. [c]All other services include nutrition and social work services.

Figure 2. Service Types Provided at Veterans Health Administration (VHA)-Operated and Contracted Community-Based Outpatient Clinics (CBOC), Fiscal Year 2016.

Table 2. Average Expenditures per Encounter by Veterans Health Administration (VHA)-Operated and Contracted Community-Based Outpatient Clinics (CBOC), Fiscal Years 2014 – 2016

Fiscal year	VHA-Operated	Contracted
2014	$219	$209
2015	$225	$218
2016	$240	$229

Source: GAO analysis of VHA data. | GAO-18-375.

Notes: Expenditures are not adjusted for inflation.

As of September 30, 2016, there were 733 CBOCs—632 VHA-operated and 101 contracted. For these analyses, data were missing for 46 CBOCs; VHA only recorded data for these clinics at the Department of Veterans Affairs medical center level. Therefore, we analyzed data for 687 CBOCs— 589 VHA-operated and 98 contracted. Further, 24 of the 687 CBOCs included in our analysis did not have 3 full fiscal years of data because they were new clinics that began operating during the time period of our review; we included data that were available.

VHA defines an encounter as a professional contact between a patient and a practitioner vested with responsibility for diagnosing, evaluating, and treating the patient's condition. Encounters can occur in both the outpatient and inpatient settings, and can include face-to-face interactions or those accomplished through telecommunications technology.

VHA pays contracted CBOCs a capitated per-member per-month rate that combines both direct and indirect expenditures, which cannot be separated from one another in VHA's managerial cost accounting system, unlike for VHA-operated CBOCs. Therefore, we examined total expenditures, which include both direct and indirect expenditures. For the VHA-operated CBOCs, we did not evaluate the methodology used by VHA to allocate indirect expenditures.

VHA-Operated CBOCs Had Higher Expenditures than Contracted CBOCs

We also found that per-encounter expenditures for almost all service types were higher on average for VHA-operated CBOCs than contracted CBOCs in fiscal year 2016; the exception was mental health care services, where VHA-operated clinics' per-encounter expenditures were 2 percent lower than for contracted clinics. The difference in per-encounter expenditures was greatest for specialty care services. For example, VHA-operated clinics' per-encounter expenditures for specialty care services were 46 percent higher than for contracted clinics.

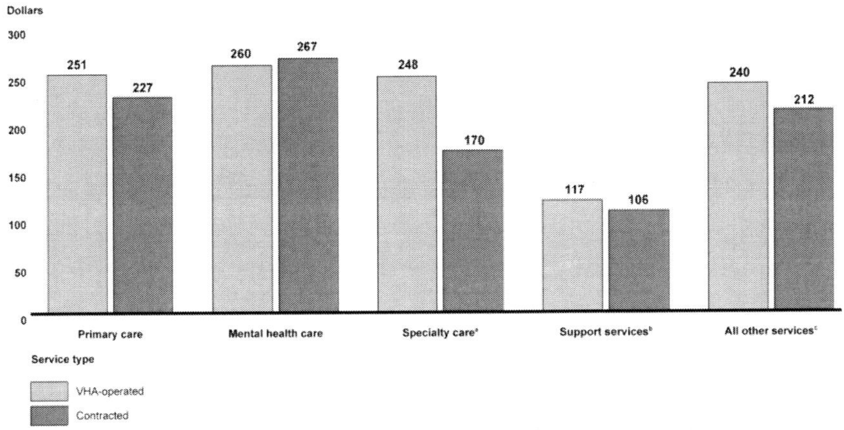

Source: GAO analysis of VHA data. | GAO-18-375.

Notes: Expenditures are not adjusted for inflation.

As of September 30, 2016, there were 733 CBOCs—632 VHA-operated and 101 contracted. For these analyses, data were missing for 46 CBOCs; VHA only recorded data for these clinics at the Department of Veterans Affairs medical center level. Therefore, we analyzed data for 687 CBOCs— 589 VHA-operated and 98 contracted.

VHA defines an encounter as a professional contact between a patient and a practitioner vested with responsibility for diagnosing, evaluating, and treating the patient's condition. Encounters can occur in both the outpatient and inpatient settings, and can include face-to-face interactions or those accomplished through telecommunications technology.

VHA pays contracted CBOCs a capitated per-member per-month rate that combines both direct and indirect expenditures, which cannot be separated from one another in VHA's managerial cost accounting system, unlike for VHA-operated CBOCs. Therefore, we examined total expenditures, which include both direct and indirect expenditures. For the VHA-operated CBOCs, we did not evaluate the methodology used by VHA to allocate indirect expenditures.

[a]Specialty care services include cardiology, gastroenterology, and rehabilitation services (e.g., physical therapy).

[b]Support services include radiology and laboratory services. [c]All other services include nutrition and social work services.

Figure 3. Veterans Health Administration (VHA)-Operated and Contracted Community-Based Outpatient Clinics (CBOC) Average per-Encounter Expenditures by Service Type, Fiscal Year 2016.

This is in contrast to primary care, where VHA-operated clinics had 11 percent higher per-encounter expenditures, on average, compared to contracted clinics. (See Figure 3.) Officials told us that several factors can influence per-encounter expenditures, including (1) differences in provider compensation and types of providers (physicians vs. physician assistants); (2) the number of patients with complex health conditions that generally require longer visits and more costly services (as opposed to patients with well-managed conditions); and (3) geographic differences in the cost of providing care. One of our selected contracted CBOCs had one of the highest per-encounter expenditures for fiscal year 2016 among all clinics. Officials from this clinic's VAMC told us this was due to the contractor being able to command a very high payment rate at the time of the contract award, due to temporarily strong local economic conditions, as well as being the only contractor in the area capable of providing the required services. Officials said the VAMC is in the process of awarding a new contract for this clinic.

Although per-encounter expenditures were generally lower for contracted CBOCs, officials from the VISNs and VAMCs in our review told us they consider several factors in determining whether a new clinic will be VHA operated or contracted. Such factors include the ability to directly monitor performance and implement new standards of care, as well as the ability to recruit and staff the clinic. For example, officials from two VAMCs in our review told us that VHA-operated clinics can be easier to manage because the VAMC has direct control of the clinic. Officials said this makes it easier to implement changes to VHA standards of care without the need to enter into contract modification negotiations. On the other hand, officials from three of the four VISNs and three of the four VAMCs in our review told us that contractors can be more flexible than VHA in recruiting staff (such as the ability to offer higher salaries), making a contracted clinic desirable for geographic areas where VHA has challenges recruiting or retaining providers.

VHA Has Not Fully Implemented Policy Requirements, and Inaccurate Information Limits Its Oversight of CBOC Quality of Care

VHA Has Not Fully Implemented CBOC Oversight Policy Requirements

We found that VHA has implemented certain oversight requirements, but not others described in Directive 1229—its policy that outlines VHA's oversight responsibilities for outpatient sites of care, including CBOCs.[23] In terms of the oversight requirements that VHA implemented, we found it has provided reports on patient satisfaction to VISNs and VAMCs on a monthly basis. Specifically, VHA distributes the results of the VHA Survey of Healthcare Experiences, a monthly survey of veterans' satisfaction with the care they received through VHA health care facilities. In addition, VHA implemented the requirement to make measures related to evaluating the progress of outpatient sites of care, such as data on wait times, workload, and costs, available on an internal VHA website. However, VHA has not implemented other oversight requirements, which is inconsistent with federal standards for internal control related to monitoring, which state that management should establish and operate monitoring activities to monitor the internal control system and evaluate the results.[24]

We found that VHA has not implemented the following requirements in Directive 1229:

- VHA has not developed guidelines for monitoring the quality and comprehensiveness of care in CBOCs. Officials from the three VHA offices with responsibility for collaborating to develop guidelines for monitoring the quality and comprehensiveness of care in CBOCs, as required in the policy, told us that they are not currently developing these guidelines and they have no plans to do

---

[23] VHA Directive 1229.

[24] GAO-14-704G.

so. First, officials from the office of the Assistant Deputy Under Secretary for Health for Policy and Planning told us they had not developed these guidelines because they no longer believed it was their office's responsibility, despite the fact that officials from the office had helped to develop the recently issued policy. Second, officials from the office of the Deputy Under Secretary for Health for Organizational Excellence told us that their office was not responsible for addressing the broader issue of monitoring clinics. Third, officials from the office of the Deputy Under Secretary for Health for Operations and Management told us that although they do not have formal guidelines in place, they believe their office meets the Directive 1229 requirement as part of their regular VISN oversight. Officials said they collect and review VISNlevel performance data, such as patient satisfaction data, which can be broken down to the level of the CBOC if there is a performance problem. However, VHA may miss clinic performance problems that are not identifiable in the VISN-level data. In addition, without developing such guidelines, VHA has not established standardized processes for how it monitors CBOCs, which can lead to inconsistent oversight. This poses the risk that veterans may be subject to different standards of care depending on the clinic visited.

- VISNs do not conduct continuous quality monitoring of CBOCs to ensure that consistent, quality care is being delivered. We found that three of the four VISNs in our review largely delegated oversight of the CBOCs to the VAMCs, rather than conducting continuous quality monitoring as required in the policy. Specifically, officials from these VISNs said that they largely focus their oversight on the VAMCs and do not separately review the performance of every CBOC unless the VAMC informs them of a quality problem at a particular clinic. Officials from the remaining VISN in our review said they do conduct CBOC-specific oversight activities. Specifically, this VISN had created a performance review survey tool that it sends to each clinic on an annual basis, and the results are reviewed by a workgroup made up of VISN staff. The workgroup examines trends across the CBOCs, including a comparison of VHA-operated and contracted performance. For example, one question in the tool asks how an individual CBOC's performance compares with others overseen by the VAMC. The delegation of oversight responsibility for the CBOCs to the VAMCs without consistent VISN-level oversight creates the potential for inconsistencies in oversight, which does not align with VHA policy to provide one standard of care for all clinics. Consequently, veterans may be subject to different standards of care across clinics.

- The Deputy Under Secretary for Health for Operations and Management has not reviewed CBOC performance with VISNs as part of the quarterly VISN performance reviews. The Deputy Under Secretary for Health for Operations and Management is responsible for conducting reviews of VISN performance with each VISN director. Specifically, the office of the Deputy Under Secretary for Health for Operations and Management is required by VHA policy to review CBOC-level performance data during quarterly VISN performance reviews. However, officials from this office and two of the VISNs we contacted told us they do not specifically do this unless the VISN identifies a performance problem. Of the remaining two VISNs, officials at one VISN reported only having mid-year and year-end meetings with VHA central office at which they did not specifically discuss the CBOCs, and officials from the other VISN said they did not have any regular quarterly performance reviews with VHA central office. This lack of consistent oversight poses the risk that VHA is not providing one, high quality standard of care to veterans across CBOCs.

VHA's CBOC Report Lacks Accurate and Complete Information

Directive 1229 requires VHA to provide reports to the VISNs and VAMCs on CBOC quality of care on a quarterly and year-end basis. We found that the CBOC Report, which is VHA's only report that allows for comparing clinical quality of care data across VHA-operated and contracted CBOCs, lacks accurate and complete information.[25] These gaps limit the CBOC Report's usefulness as a monitoring tool to determine whether VHA-operated and contracted CBOCs are providing the same standard of care. This is inconsistent with federal standards for internal control for information and communication, which state that management should use quality information to achieve the entity's objectives.[26]

Specifically, VHA distributes the CBOC Report to VISNs and VAMCs on a quarterly and year-end basis, which compiles CBOC quality of care performance results based on the Healthcare Effectiveness Data and Information Set (HEDIS)—an industry standard set of quality measures.[27] VISNs and VAMCs have access to other types of CBOC performance data, such as patient satisfaction data and wait time data, but these data are not used to assess clinical quality of care and they cannot be used to examine performance across all CBOCs or stratified by VHA-operated versus contracted CBOCs. In contrast, the CBOC Report allows for the comparison of clinical quality of care data across all CBOCs, which can be stratified according to whether the clinic is VHA-operated or contracted.

However, we found the following issues with the CBOC Report:

---

[25] The CBOC Report is prepared and distributed by VHA's Reporting, Analytics, Performance, Improvements and Development office within the office of the Deputy Under Secretary for Health for Organizational Excellence.

[26] GAO-14-704G.

[27] HEDIS is a standardized dataset designed by the National Committee for Quality Assurance—a private, nonprofit organization—to help consumers compare the performance of health plans in providing selected services. VHA has adopted HEDIS measures to assess the quality of care provided by facilities in the VHA health care system. These measures include those related to behavioral health screening, diabetes, and heart disease.

- **Incorrect classification of CBOCs.** We compared CBOCs from the most recent CBOC Report at the time of our review (the first quarter of fiscal year 2017) against sites in the VAST system as of January 3, 2017, which is VHA's listing of all VHA sites of care and their characteristics. We found that 22 percent of sites were incorrectly classified as CBOCs, based on the site classifications in VAST. Several of these sites were much more complex, such as health care centers and VAMCs.[28] For example, a VAMC was included in the report as a CBOC, but this VAMC has three specialized intensive care units and serves as a regional referral center for intensive inpatient surgery, including open heart surgery. In addition, we also identified sites included in the report that provided less complex services than those that are provided in CBOCs, such as other outpatient services sites.
- VHA officials who produce the CBOC Report told us that, prior to the establishment of the VAST site classifications in 2014, they used their judgment to classify existing sites of care as CBOCs and they have not updated their classifications since then.[29] For sites established since 2014, officials told us they use the VAST site classifications, but may also use their judgment in certain situations. For example, if a site's classification changed in VAST from a non-CBOC to a CBOC, they would make a decision about whether to classify it as a CBOC in the report by examining various aspects of the facility, such as the services provided and encounters. This procedure differs from what is documented in the methodology section of the CBOC Report, which states that site classifications are based on VAST. Further, VHA officials said they did not have a document available that outlined how they make these decisions. Because the site classifications in the CBOC Report are based, in part, on officials' judgment in addition to the classifications in VAST, the report does not present accurate

[28] Health care centers and VAMCs are, in general, highly complex and provide services that are much more resource-intensive than the services that are provided in CBOCs.

[29] VHA Handbook 1006.02.

information on CBOCs across VHA and is of limited usefulness to VHA as a tool to ensure that VHA-operated and contracted CBOCs are providing the same standard of care that is of high quality.

- Missing CBOCs. We found that 53 CBOCs (7 percent of all CBOCs) were missing from the CBOC Report from the first quarter of fiscal year 2017, rendering the data incomplete. VHA officials provided examples of why a CBOC might not be included in the report. For example, a newer CBOC might not be included because it did not have quality of care data available at the time the report was developed. However, we identified several other sites that were listed in the report, despite unavailable data.
- Inaccurate summary calculations. Due to the incorrect site classifications and missing CBOCs, the national- and VISN-level summary calculations of performance in the CBOC Report were also inaccurate. Specifically, the report includes national- and VISN-level averages for each HEDIS measure, which VHA officials can use as benchmarks for clinic performance. These averages were overinclusive—incorporating performance results from additional sites that were not CBOCs, and under-inclusive—omitting performance results from CBOCs that were missing from the report. These inaccuracies may lead VHA officials to draw incorrect conclusions about the quality of care provided in CBOCs. For example, officials from one VAMC told us that they use the national averages as benchmarks against which they compare the performance of their CBOCs. Because this VAMC requires CBOCs with lower-than-average HEDIS performance results to develop a formal action plan to improve performance, officials may not be identifying clinics that are in need of an action plan due to the inaccuracy of the averages. In addition, VHA central office officials who develop the CBOC Report said that the results from recent reports have shown that VHA-operated and contracted clinics in general provided the same standard of care, but this conclusion may not be correct as it is based on unreliable data.

- No guidance or training for use of the CBOC Report. VHA central office officials do not provide guidance or training specific to the CBOC Report to assist VISNs and VAMCs in using it to oversee CBOCs. This is inconsistent with federal standards for internal control related to the control environment, which state that management should, among other things, develop personnel to achieve the entity's objectives. Such development may include training to enable individuals to develop competencies appropriate for key roles.[30] In our review of the CBOC Report from the first quarter of fiscal year 2017, we found that in several places in the report, shorthand text and acronyms were used, but not defined. In addition, although there is a methodology section, it is not clear that the measures described in the report are HEDIS measures, for which VHA makes training available. Several VAMC and VISN officials stated that guidance or training that is specific to understanding the CBOC Report would be helpful. If VISNs and VAMCs are not trained on how to use the report, they may not know how to use it to oversee CBOCs and ensure they are providing one standard of care that is of high quality.
- No requirement for VISNs or VAMCs to use the CBOC Report. VHA does not require that the CBOC Report be used as a tool to oversee CBOCs. As a result, we found that the report was not widely used. Specifically, an official from the office of the Deputy Under Secretary for Health for Organizational Excellence—which produces the CBOC Report—told us that the office's role is to compile the reports and distribute them, but not to monitor performance. Officials from the office of the Deputy Under Secretary for Health for Operations and Management said that VISNs and VAMCs are expected to use the report as part of their CBOC oversight; however, we found there is no requirement that they do so. We found that officials from three of the four VISNs and three of the four VAMCs in our review were not regularly

[30] GAO-14-704G.

using the CBOC Report. Officials from one of the four VAMCs and one of the four VISNs in our review were using it as part of CBOC oversight activities at the time of our review. Officials from another VISN said that they planned to start using the CBOC Report after we made them aware of it during our interview. If VISN and VAMC officials do not use the report as a part of their oversight, they may be missing opportunities to compare VHA-operated and contracted CBOCs and ensure they are providing one standard of care that is of high quality.

CONCLUSION

CBOCs are an integral part of VHA's health care delivery system, and VHA requires that such clinics, whether VHA-operated or contracted, provide the same standard of care to veterans that is of high quality. Although VHA has implemented certain policy requirements for CBOC oversight, we found several weaknesses in its oversight that make it difficult to determine whether it is ensuring this consistent standard of care across the clinics.

Specifically, VHA has not fully implemented oversight requirements that align with its established policies, including a requirement to establish guidelines for overseeing CBOC quality of care. The CBOC Report, as VHA's only report comparing clinical quality of care across both VHA-operated and contracted clinics, could be an important part of those guidelines. However, as it currently stands, the report is inaccurate and incomplete and VISNs and VAMCs are not trained on or required to use it; thus, it is of limited use to VHA, including the VISNs and VAMCs that have responsibility for CBOC oversight. As a result, VHA lacks assurance that both VHA-operated and contracted CBOCs are providing one standard of care that is of high quality.

Recommendations for Executive Action

We are making the following four recommendations to the VHA Undersecretary for Health:

Implement oversight requirements that align with VHA's existing policy, including developing guidelines for monitoring quality of care in CBOCs. (Recommendation 1)

Establish a process for regularly updating the CBOC Report to ensure it contains an accurate and complete list of CBOCs that is consistent with VHA's established site classifications. (Recommendation 2)

Ensure that VISNs and VAMCs receive guidance or training on how to use the CBOC Report. (Recommendation 3)

Require the use of the CBOC Report as an oversight tool for ensuring one standard of care that is of high quality across VHA-operated and contracted CBOCs. (Recommendation 4)

Agency Comments

We provided VA with a draft of this chapter for its review and comment. VA provided written comments, which are reprinted in appendix I. In its written comments, VA concurred with all four of the report's recommendations, and identified actions it is taking to implement them.

We are sending copies of this chapter to the appropriate congressional committees, the Acting Secretary of Veterans Affairs, the Under Secretary for Health, and other interested parties.

Debra A. Draper
Director, Health Care

List of Requesters

The Honorable Johnny Isakson
Chairman

The Honorable Jon Tester
Ranking Member
Committee on Veterans' Affairs
United States Senate

The Honorable Phil Roe
Chairman

The Honorable Tim Walz
Ranking Member
Committee on Veterans' Affairs
House of Representatives

The Honorable Derek Kilmer
House of Representatives

The Honorable Mark Takano
House of Representatives

APPENDIX I: COMMENTS FROM THE DEPARTMENT OF VETERANS AFFAIRS

DEPARTMENT OF VETERANS AFFAIRS
WASHINGTON DC 20420

March 19, 2018

Ms. Debra Draper
Director
Health Care
U.S. Government Accountability Office
441 G Street, NW
Washington, DC 20548

Dear Ms. Draper:

The Department of Veterans Affairs (VA) has reviewed the Government Accountability Office's (GAO) draft report, ***"VA HEALTH CARE: Actions Needed to Improve Oversight of Community-Based Outpatient Clinics"*** (GAO-18-375).

The enclosure sets forth the actions to be taken to address the GAO draft report recommendations.

VA appreciates the opportunity to comment on your draft report.

Sincerely,

Jacquelyn Hayes-Byrd
Deputy Chief of Staff

Department of Veterans Affairs (VA) Comments to
Government Accountability Office (GAO) Draft Report
VA HEALTH CARE: Actions Needed to Improve Oversight of Community-Based Outpatient Clinics
(GAO-18-375)

<u>Recommendation 1</u>: Implement oversight requirements that align with VHA's existing policy, including developing guidelines for monitoring quality of care in CBOCs.

<u>VA Comment</u>: Concur. In collaboration with the Office of Performance Measurement in the Office of Reporting, Analytics, Performance, Improvement and Deployment, the Office of the Assistant Deputy Under Secretary for Health for Clinical Operations will issue guidance outlining requirements for Veterans Integrated Service Networks (VISN) and VA medical facilities. These requirements will be discussed with Network Directors, Medical Center Directors, and Chief Medical Officers on various Veterans Health Administration (VHA) National calls. Additionally, the Deputy Under Secretary for Health for Operations and Management (DUSHOM) will incorporate these requirements into the quarterly VISN Director Performance reviews. The status is in process with a target completion date of September 2018.

<u>Recommendation 2</u>: Establish a process for regularly updating the CBOC Report to ensure it contains an accurate and complete list of CBOCs that is consistent with VHA's established site classifications.

<u>VA Comment</u>: Concur. The Office of the Deputy Under Secretary for Health for Operations and Management will develop a process for regularly updating the VA Site Tracking application to ensure the Community-Based Outpatient Clinic (CBOC) Report accurately reflects requests received by the VHA Support Service Center from VA medical facilities. The status is in process with a target completion date of September 2018.

<u>Recommendation 3</u>: Ensure that VISNs and VAMCs receive guidance or training on how to use the CBOC Report.

<u>VA Comment</u>: Concur. The Office of the Assistant Deputy Under Secretary for Health for Clinical Operations will provide guidance concerning use of the CBOC Report to VISNs' Chief Medical and Quality Management Officers. Additionally, in collaboration with the Office of Performance Measurement in the Office of Reporting, Analytics, Performance, Improvement and Deployment, the Office of the Deputy Under Secretary for Health for Operations and Management will provide training to VA medical facilities during the annual training on the Performance Measure report. The status is in process with a target completion date of September 2018.

<u>Recommendation 4</u>: Require the use of the CBOC Report as an oversight tool for ensuring one standard of care that is of high-quality across VHA-operated and contracted CBOCs.

<u>VA Comment</u>: Concur. The Office of the Assistant Deputy Under Secretary for Health for Clinical Operations will provide guidance concerning use of the CBOC Report to VISNs Chief Medical and Quality Management Officers. Additionally, in collaboration with the Office of Performance Measurement in the Office of Reporting, Analytics, Performance, Improvement and Deployment, DUSHOM will provide training to VA medical facilities during the annual training on the Performance Measure report. The DUSHOM will also incorporate the required utilization into the quarterly VISN Director Performance reviews. The status is in process with a target completion date of September 2018.

In: Improvements Needed in the VA ... ISBN: 978-1-53615-971-4
Editor: Charles Copeland

Chapter 9

PHARMACY INVENTORY MANAGEMENT COULD BENEFIT FROM SYSTEM-WIDE OVERSIGHT*

United States Government Accountability Office

ABBREVIATIONS

GS	general schedule
IT	information technology
NAC	National Acquisition Center
OIT	Office of Information and Technology
PBM	Pharmacy Benefits Management Service
VA	Department of Veterans Affairs
VACO	VA Central Office
VAMC	VA Medical Center
VA OIG	VA Office of Inspector General

---

* This is an edited, reformatted and augmented version of United States Government Accountability Office; Report to the Subcommittee on Oversight and Investigations, Committee on Veterans' Affairs, House of Representatives, Publication No. GAO-18-658, dated September 2018.

VISN	Veterans Integrated Service Network
VistA	Veterans Health Information Systems and Technology Architecture
VPE	VISN Pharmacy Executive

WHY GAO DID THIS STUDY

VA provides health care services, including pharmacy services, to approximately 9 million veterans each year. Since 2000, VAMCs have faced recurring challenges in managing their pharmacy inventories, including difficulties with accurately accounting for and updating inventory totals through their pharmacy systems.

GAO was asked to review VA pharmacy inventory management. This chapter (1) describes approaches selected VAMCs use to manage their pharmacy inventories and (2) assesses the extent to which VA oversees VAMCs' efforts to manage their pharmacy inventories.

To conduct this work, GAO visited a non-generalizable selection of five VAMCs chosen for the complexity of services offered and variation in location. GAO also reviewed VA national policies and local polices for the selected VAMCs and interviewed VA officials at the headquarters, regional, and local levels. GAO assessed VA's oversight of pharmacy management in the context of federal internal control standards.

WHAT GAO RECOMMENDS

GAO recommends that VA designate a focal point for overseeing VAMCs' pharmacy inventory management efforts system-wide and define the focal point's responsibilities. VA concurred in principle with the recommendation.

WHAT GAO FOUND

Selected Department of Veterans Affairs' (VA) medical centers (VAMC) use generally similar approaches for managing their pharmacy inventories. For example, all VAMCs store certain medications in secured areas. However, GAO found that VAMCs have also taken unique approaches for procuring and tracking medications, as allowed under VA policy. For example, to better address medication shortages, one VAMC pharmacy GAO visited established a shortage committee that meets on a weekly basis. Another VAMC pharmacy uses an automated dispensing machine together with compatible software that allows the pharmacy to track the location of most inpatient medications in real-time (see figure 3).

GAO also found that VA's oversight of VAMCs' pharmacy inventory management is limited as VA lacks a comprehensive inventory management system or a focal point for system-wide oversight. In May 2018, VA signed a contract for a new electronic health records system that should allow VA to monitor VAMCs' inventories; however, VA officials expect implementation of this system to take up to 10 years. Based on a review of VA policies and interviews with VA officials, GAO found that VA has not designated a focal point with defined responsibilities for system-wide oversight of VAMCs' pharmacy inventory management. This is inconsistent with federal internal control standards for monitoring and establishing structure and authority to achieve an entity's objectives. Without a focal point for system-wide oversight, VA has limited awareness of the unique approaches that VAMCs use to manage their inventories and is missing an opportunity to evaluate these approaches. Additionally, VA cannot effectively share and standardize inventory management best practices as appropriate. Having a focal point is especially important given that VAMCs have historically had challenges in managing their inventories and a comprehensive pharmacy inventory management system may not be available for the foreseeable future.

September 27, 2018

The Honorable Jack Bergman
Chairman

The Honorable Ann Kuster
Ranking Member
Subcommittee on Oversight and Investigations
Committee on Veterans' Affairs
House of Representatives

The Department of Veterans Affairs (VA) provides health care services, including pharmacy services, to approximately 9 million veterans each year.[1] Veterans can receive a range of services at the approximately 170 VA medical centers (VAMC) throughout the nation, including traditional hospital-based services such as surgery, critical care, and mental health care. As a significant part of delivering health care to veterans, VAMCs also provide medications, prescription refills, and other pharmacy services.[2] These VAMCs are generally responsible for managing their own pharmacy inventories—that is, for procuring, storing, tracking, and dispensing medications to veterans.

Managing pharmacy inventories effectively to provide pharmacy services to veterans can be challenging. In 2000, a VA Office of Inspector General (OIG) audit found that VAMC pharmacies carried excess inventory due to a reliance on informal inventory methods and identified the need for VAMCs to use modern inventory techniques and automated pharmacy inventory management systems.[3] Subsequent OIG and GAO reports have identified some of the technological challenges VA faces in overseeing its VAMC pharmacies. For example, a 2009 VA OIG report found that VA could not accurately account for the medications at VAMC

[1] The VA administers its health care services through the Veterans Health Administration.

[2] Veterans may also receive prescribed medications through VA's mail delivery service provided by seven consolidated outpatient mail pharmacy facilities or, when needed, by mail from VAMC pharmacies.

[3] Department of Veterans Affairs, Office of Inspector General, *Audit of VA Medical Center Management of Pharmaceutical Inventories*, 99-00186-86 (Washington, D.C.: June 30, 2000).

pharmacies because VA lacked reliable information to do so.[4] Similarly, in 2017 we reported that VA does not have the systems that would allow it to keep a perpetual inventory and monitor VAMC pharmacy inventory levels in real time.[5] These reports have raised broader concerns about how VA oversees its VAMCs' pharmacies.

You asked us to review the management and oversight of VAMC pharmacy inventories. In this chapter, we

- describe how selected VAMCs manage their pharmacy inventories; and
- assess the extent to which VA oversees VAMCs' efforts to manage their pharmacy inventories.

To describe how selected VAMCs manage their pharmacy inventories, we identified their approaches for procuring, storing, tracking, dispensing, and disposing of medications, the main process that all pharmacies generally use to manage their pharmacy inventories. Our review focused on pharmacy inventory of all medications—including controlled and non-controlled substances—dispensed within the VAMCs' inpatient wards or at their outpatient pharmacies.[6] Our review focused on VAMCs' management of their inpatient and outpatient pharmacy inventories; as such we did not review pharmacy inventory management at the consolidated mail

---

[4] Department of Veterans Affairs, Office of Inspector General, *Audit of Veterans Health Administration's Management of Non-Controlled Drugs*, 08-01322-114 (Washington, D.C.: June 23, 2009).

[5] GAO, *VA Information Technology: Pharmacy System Needs Additional Capabilities for Viewing, Exchanging, and Using Data to Better Serve Veterans,* GAO-17-179 (Washington, D.C.: June 14, 2017).

[6] According to the Controlled Substances Act, as amended, the term "controlled substance" means "a drug or other substance, or immediate precursor, included in [one of five classification schedules]." A controlled substance is placed in a respective schedule based on whether it has a currently accepted medical use in treatment in the United States and its relative abuse potential and likelihood of causing dependence. Examples of controlled substances include pain relievers, such as Percocet or OxyContin, as well as tranquilizers, stimulants, and sedatives available only by prescription. Pub. L. No. 91-513, §§ 102, 201-02, 84 Stat. 1236, 1243, 1245-52 (1970) (codified as amended at 21 U.S.C. §§ 802, 811-812); 21 C.F.R. Parts 1300 and 1308 (2018).

outpatient pharmacies.[7] We conducted site visits at a non-generalizable sample of five VAMCs that we selected based on diversity in geographic regions, differences in facility complexity, and variation in pharmacy operations efficiency determined by comparing expected and observed pharmacy expenditures by VAMC for fiscal year 2016.[8] Although VA officials identified limitations in the pharmacy expenditures data, we found that the data were sufficiently reliable to use as one criterion for selecting VAMCs to visit.[9] The five VAMCs we visited are located in Cheyenne, Wyoming; Danville, Illinois; Philadelphia, Pennsylvania; Richmond, Virginia; and San Francisco, California. At each of these five VAMCs, we toured inpatient and outpatient pharmacy operations and conducted semi-structured interviews with VAMC officials and staff responsible for managing pharmacy inventory—including VAMC Executives, the Chief and Associate Chief of Pharmacy Services, pharmacy staff, and nursing staff. We also observed the information technology (IT) systems and automated medication dispensing machines and software that each VAMC uses to manage pharmacy inventory. In addition, we reviewed relevant national VA and local VAMC policies and guidance for managing pharmacy inventory.

---

[7] According to the Veterans Health Administration, outpatient prescribing is performed most predominantly, with the consolidated mail outpatient pharmacies providing approximately 80 percent of all outpatient prescriptions to veterans. For fiscal year 2016, the Veterans Health Administration reported that it provided outpatient pharmacy services to approximately 5 million veterans. The agency further reported that about 31 million outpatient prescriptions were filled at VAMC and outpatient clinic pharmacies, and about 116 million prescriptions were filled by consolidated mail outpatient pharmacies.

[8] VA assigns each VAMC a complexity score based upon patient population served, clinical services offered, education and research complexity, and administrative complexity. Specifically, each VAMC is assigned a score between 1 and 3 (level 1 is broken down further into 1a, 1b, and 1c), with level 1 being the most complex, using a facility complexity model.

[9] This expenditure data is a compilation of statistical models and measures designed to help VAMCs monitor pharmacy expenditures and identify areas for improvement. However, according to VA officials, one flaw of the data is that they make assumptions that are not fully representative of the patient population.

To examine the extent to which VA oversees VAMCs' efforts to manage their pharmacy inventories, we assessed the extent to which VA Central Office (VACO) and the Veterans Integrated Service Networks (VISN) oversee the five selected VAMCs' management of pharmacy inventory. The VISNs report to VACO and are responsible for managing and overseeing VAMCs within their geographic area. To conduct our work, we reviewed VA policies, procedures, and guidance pertaining to the management and oversight of pharmacy inventory to determine the extent of VACO's and the VISNs' oversight responsibilities. This included a review of meeting minutes from regularly scheduled calls between VACO and VISN officials. We also interviewed VACO officials from the Pharmacy Benefits Management Service (PBM), the National Acquisition Center (NAC), and the Office of Information and Technology (OIT) to determine their roles in overseeing VAMC pharmacy inventory. In addition, we interviewed the five VISN Pharmacy Executives (VPE) responsible for assisting the selected VAMCs with pharmacy-related tasks. We examined VA's oversight in the context of federal standards for internal controls related to establishing structure and authority to achieve the entity's objectives and internal controls related to monitoring.[10] To better understand other integrated health systems' best practices for managing pharmacy inventory, we also interviewed representatives from the American Society of Health-System Pharmacists, the Mayo Clinic, and the Cleveland Clinic. We also reviewed our previous work and the VA OIG's work that is related to VAMC's pharmacy inventory management.

We conducted this performance audit from September 2017 to September 2018 in accordance with generally accepted government auditing standards. Those standards require that we plan and perform the audit to obtain sufficient, appropriate evidence to provide a reasonable basis for our findings and conclusions based on our audit objectives. We believe that the evidence obtained provides a reasonable basis for our findings and conclusions based on our audit objectives.

---

[10] GAO, *Standards for Internal Control in the Federal Government,* GAO-14-704G (Washington, D.C.: September 2014).

BACKGROUND

General Process for Managing Pharmacy Inventories in Hospital Settings

In general, the process for managing inventories of medications at VAMCs and non-VA pharmacies in hospital settings is similar. The steps of the process are (1) procuring medications from vendors or other suppliers, (2) receiving and storing medications, (3) tracking medications to account for all items and prevent diversion, (4) dispensing medications to patients, and (5) disposing of expired or wasted medications. Hospital settings include both inpatient and outpatient pharmacies.

Procurement

Pharmacies use a procurement process to order medications for pharmacy inventory, which includes activities such as medication selection, cost analysis, purchasing procedures, and record keeping. As part of medication selection, pharmacies may use a formulary, which is a list of medications that have been approved for prescription within a hospital or health care system.

A prime vendor or wholesaler is one of the most commonly used sources to obtain medications for the pharmacy. Prime vendors order large quantities of medications from manufacturers, allowing pharmacies to purchase various products from many drug manufacturers at once. Orders for products that are not carried by the prime vendor may need to be ordered through another source, such as directly from the manufacturer.

Receipt and Storage

When medications are delivered to the pharmacy, staff are to take several steps to properly receive and store the shipment. For example, to ensure there is segregation of duties, the person responsible for ordering and purchasing the medications is supposed to be different than the person receiving and stocking pharmacy inventory. Additionally, any delivered products that require special storage conditions, such as freezing or refrigeration, are to be checked in first to maintain the stability of the medication.

Tracking

Once in storage, pharmacies use a variety of tools to account for the filling, dispensing, and removal of medications in both inpatient and outpatient settings. Some pharmacies have software that allows them to track inventory in real time, an ability known as maintaining perpetual inventory. A perpetual inventory system is a method of recording the quantity of a particular medication continuously as prescriptions are filled and dispensed. After each prescription is filled and dispensed to the patient, the amount of medication used for the prescription is removed from the inventory to ensure the quantity on hand recorded by the software is always current.

Many medications have barcodes on their packaging to allow for easy identification of the medication in a computer system. The barcode generally includes the product's National Drug Code, which indicates the name and package size of the medication. In the hospital setting, medications can be scanned out of the pharmacy and into machines for storage on hospital wards.

Dispensing

In both inpatient wards and outpatient pharmacies, automated dispensing machines and barcode technology can assist staff in maintaining and dispensing medications to patients. Automated dispensing machines generally include several drawers and cabinets that have pockets or trays that hold preset levels of a variety of common medications. They may also be used to hold controlled substances, generally in locked boxes or cubes within the machine. On hospital wards medication in automated dispensing machines is often packaged in unit doses—individually packaged medications for patient use. Barcodes can help verify a prescription before nurses give medication to a patient. Hospitals that do not have automatic dispensing machines use carts with drawers filled with each patient's medication. Outpatient pharmacies use automated dispensing machines to assist with filling prescriptions. Depending on the type of automated dispensing machine, the capabilities can include label printing, pill counting, pouring pills into prescription bottles, and applying the label to the prescription bottle.

Return or Disposal

Medication waste and expired medications are to be pulled from pharmacy inventory and either returned to a reverse distributor or manufacturer for credit or, if not eligible for return, disposed of by the pharmacy or sent to an outside company for destruction.[11]

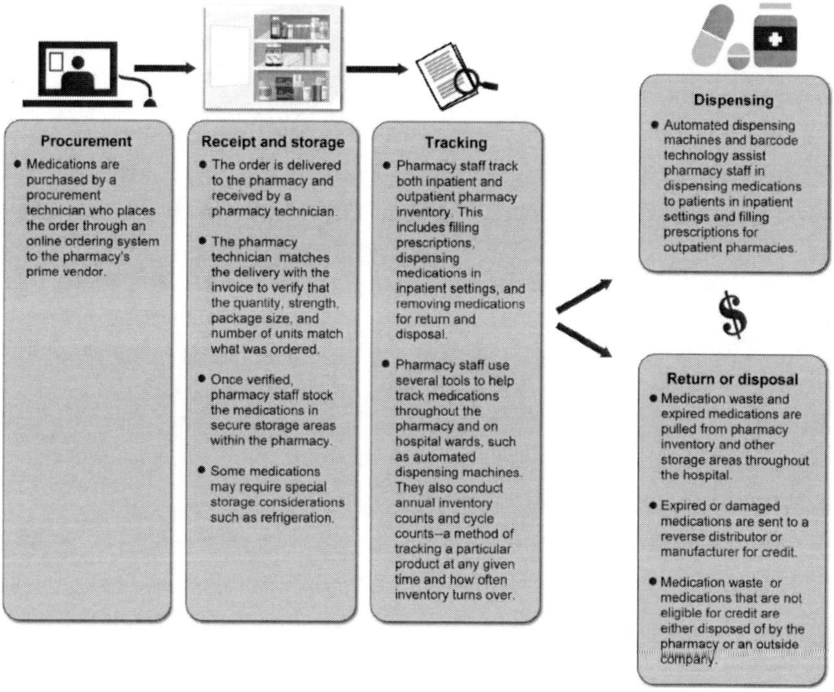

Source: GAO analysis of Industry guidelines for inventory management. | GAO-18-658.

Figure 1. Pharmacy Inventory Management Process within a Hospital Setting.

---

[11] Reverse distributors are companies that take back expired, recalled, or damaged medications from pharmacies and complete the necessary paperwork required by each manufacturer to receive credit for returned items.

Reverse distributors charge a fee, which is generally a percentage of the refund that is automatically deducted from the final refund amount.

Figure 1 provides an overview of the steps of the pharmacy inventory management process.

VA Organizational Structure and Pharmacy Policies

VA's health care system is organized into entities at the headquarters, regional, and local levels. At the headquarters level, PBM is responsible for supporting VISNs and VAMCs with a broad range of pharmacy services, such as promoting appropriate drug therapy, ensuring medication safety, providing clinical guidance to pharmacists and other clinicians, and maintaining VA's formulary of medications and supplies VAMCs use to deliver pharmacy benefits. VA's OIT is responsible for providing technology services across the department, including the development and management of all IT assets and resources. As such, the office supports VA's health care system in planning for and acquiring IT capabilities within VA's health care system network of hospitals, outpatient facilities, and pharmacies. VA's NAC is responsible for administering various health care-related acquisition and logistics programs across VA.

At the regional level, VAMCs are located in one of 18 VISNs. Each VISN is responsible for overseeing VAMC pharmacies within a defined geographic region. At the local level, there are approximately 170 VAMCs. Each VAMC is responsible for implementing VA's pharmacy policies and programming.

VA policy establishes parameters for VAMCs to follow when managing their pharmacy inventories. These policies address various aspects of pharmacy services, including inpatient and outpatient pharmacy services, general pharmacy requirements, supply chain management, controlled substances management, and the formulary management process. For example, the Supply Chain Inventory Management directive states that all VAMC pharmacies should use the prime vendor inventory management software to calculate the amount of each inventory item they need to reorder.[12] However, the directive also states that there are additional pharmacy inventory tools available to VAMC pharmacies and that each pharmacy has the option to use its own automated inventory management systems to generate orders for its prime vendor. VA policy does not specify minimum quantities to order; instead, VAMC procurement staff is authorized to use their expertise to determine the appropriate quantity to order.[13]

Selected VAMCs Have Generally Similar Approaches for Managing Their Pharmacy Inventories, with Some Unique Approaches

In general, all five of the selected VAMCs we reviewed take similar approaches for the various steps included in the pharmacy inventory management process—that is, procuring medications from vendors or other suppliers, receiving and storing these medications, tracking medications at the pharmacy to account for all items and prevent diversion, dispensing medications to patients, and disposing of expired medications.[14] (See Figure 2).

We found that while the five selected VAMCs have similar approaches for receiving and storing, dispensing, and disposing of medications, some VAMCs have also taken unique approaches in implementing two steps of the pharmacy inventory management process: procurement and tracking. VA policy outlines parameters for VAMCs to manage their pharmacy inventories, and VA officials told us that VAMC pharmacy staff can use discretion to implement their own approaches for managing their pharmacy inventories.

---

[12] Veterans Health Administration Directive 1761(1), *Supply Chain Inventory Management*. (Washington, D.C.: Oct. 24, 2016).

[13] VA officials also noted that there is a national rollup of inventory management orders that provides VISN officials with an opportunity to address any inventory outliers.

[14] VA is currently evaluating national contracts for a reverse distributor who would both dispose of medications and also process medication returns for credits. VA officials told us that they plan to award one contract to a small, veteran-owned business to cover VA-wide reverse distribution services by August 2018.

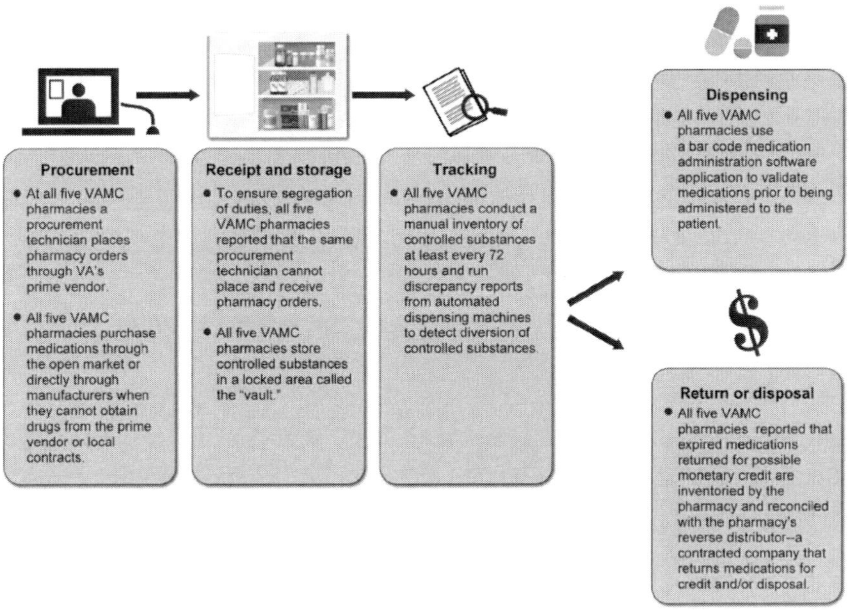

Source: GAO analysis of VA information. | GAO-18-658.

Figure 2. Similar Approaches to the Pharmacy Inventory Management Process Used by Selected Department of Veterans Affairs Medical Centers (VAMC).

Procurement

All five of the selected VAMC pharmacies we reviewed use several sources of information to inform future orders—including past purchase order history reports from VA's prime vendor, manual inventory counts by pharmacy staff, and automated dispensing machine inventory information. VA officials told us that all VAMCs also track procurement spending and its impact on the VAMCs' budget and spending. However, pharmacy officials at one of the selected VAMCs we visited told us they use VA's health information system—Veterans Health Information Systems and Technology Architecture (VistA)—and additional prime vendor reports to identify specific information regarding 1) expiring medications that may need to be re-purchased, 2) medications that account for the top 80 percent of pharmacy costs, and 3) all medications that are purchased daily.[15] VAMC officials told us these reports help them to better manage pharmacy inventory and track pharmacy spending.

To better anticipate and address potential medication shortages, officials at another selected VAMC pharmacy told us they established a shortage committee that meets on a weekly basis. Established in September 2017, the committee includes the Director of Pharmacy and other pharmacy staff. Our review of meeting notes shows that the committee discusses which medications could experience or are experiencing shortages and how the VAMC could adjust to these shortages by, for example, developing clinical and logistical solutions to help maintain optimal patient care. According to the officials at the selected VAMC pharmacy, the committee has been an effective resource to help manage pharmacy inventory problems should they occur.

Several VAMC officials also told us that the procurement technicians, who are responsible for ordering pharmacy inventory, are very important because they possess valuable institutional knowledge based on many years of experience and training.[16] However, VAMC officials told us the salaries and potential career advancement opportunities for procurement technicians can be limited, and the officials expressed concern that these technicians could find better opportunities within the VAMC or with external employers.[17] To help retain procurement technicians, two of the selected VAMC pharmacies we visited have created higher paying

[15] To enable the provision of health care services to veterans, VA uses its integrated health information system VistA. The system consists of approximately 200 separate computer applications and modules, 17 of which include pharmacy related applications.

[16] We spoke with the Chief Pharmacy Officer and pharmacy staff from Mayo Clinic who told us that procurement specialists go through intensive on-the-job training. They told us that the qualifications for inventory management procurement positions with the Mayo Clinic include a 4-year degree and previous experience, and that it takes about 2 to 3 months of intensive job training and about a full year of work experience before a procurement specialist is comfortable in the position.

[17] Challenges in recruiting and retaining staff are not unique to pharmacy operations and also affect other areas in the VA workforce. For example, in 2017 we reported that the Veterans Health Administration's financial incentives for recruiting and retaining physicians do not always result in competitive salary packages, and funding for incentives was often inadequate at the VAMC level. GAO, *Veterans Health Administration: Better Data and Evaluation Could Help Improve Physician Staffing, Recruitment, and Retention Strategies,* GAO-18-124 (Washington, D.C.: Oct.19, 2017).

procurement technician positions (General Schedule level 8 [GS-8] positions, instead of GS-6 or GS-7).[18]

Tracking

To better identify potential instances of diversion, two of the selected VAMC pharmacies use enhanced analytics software on the automated dispensing machines in their inpatient wards to track how frequently controlled substances and other frequently utilized medications are prescribed. For example, one of the pharmacies uses data from these reports to identify how often individual staff members are accessing automated dispensing machines. Additionally, officials at a third VAMC recently deployed automated dispensing machines that are equipped with an enhanced analytics program that can identify trends associated with diversion.[19] The remaining two VAMCs we visited do not have enhanced analytic software that could help them to identify instances of potential diversion.

Across all 5 selected VAMCs, we observed several different IT systems used to help manage non-controlled inpatient inventory. One of the selected VAMC pharmacies uses a modular automated dispensing machine together with inventory management software that maintains a perpetual inventory for most non-controlled substances stored in its inpatient pharmacy.[20] (See Figure 3). According to officials, this software has allowed the pharmacy to reduce waste and improve staff workflow, as staff do not have to spend time tracking down inventory. None of the other VAMC pharmacies we visited have the capability to track non-controlled substances in real time.

---

[18] The General Schedule (GS) classification and pay system covers the majority of Federal employees in professional, technical, administrative, and clerical positions. The General Schedule has 15 grades--GS-1 (lowest) to GS-15 (highest). Agencies establish the grade of each position based on the level of difficulty, responsibility, and qualifications required.

[19] In April and May of 2018, this VAMC deployed 12 new automated dispensing machines in inpatient wards with this enhanced software.

[20] Some items, such as bulk bottles, cannot be tracked in real time because the software detects bulk bottles as 1 unit and does not account for the individual pills within the bottles.

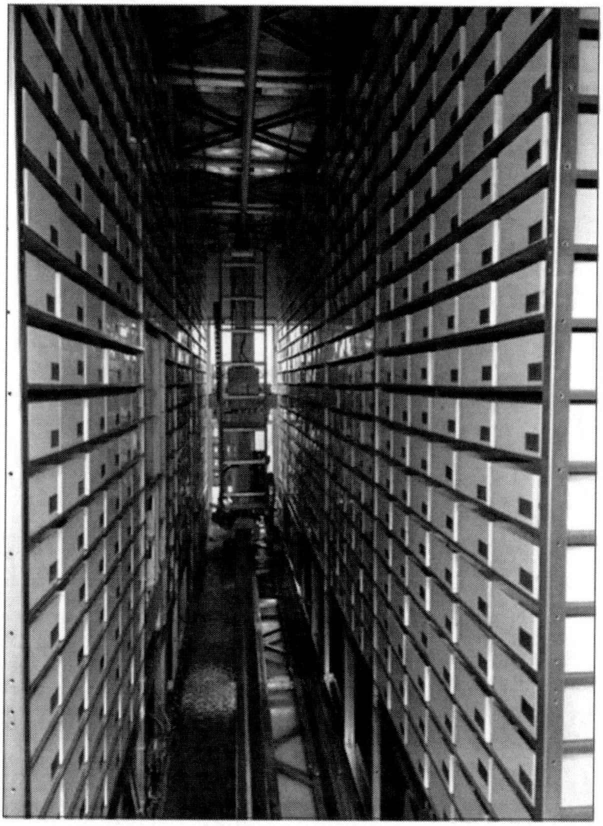

Source: Department of Veterans Affairs. | GAO-18-658.

Figure 3. Automated Medication Dispensing Machine at a Department of Veterans Affairs Medical Center.

Additionally, to more efficiently identify medication lot numbers during recalls, one VAMC pharmacy we visited was in the process of implementing a technology that allows pharmacy staff to scan a case of medication with the same national drug code, lot number, and expiration date and then print and attach a radio frequency identification tag to each medication bottle. The tag allows for quick electronic identification of the medication for disposal. Other selected VAMC pharmacies manually identify recalled medications from inventory based on the name of the medication and lot number.

Oversight of Pharmacy Inventory Management Is Limited, as VA Lacks a Comprehensive Inventory Management System or a Focal Point for System-Wide Oversight

VA does not yet have a VA-wide pharmacy inventory management system in place that would allow it to monitor VAMC pharmacy inventory in real time and provide better oversight of how VAMC pharmacies manage their inventories. We found that VACO and the five VISNs we reviewed provide some oversight related to VAMC pharmacy inventory management. However, that oversight is limited, as no entity has been assigned responsibility for overseeing system-wide performance of VAMC pharmacies in managing their inventories.

VA's Oversight of VAMCs' Pharmacy Inventory Management Is Limited, in Part Because VA Has Not Yet Implemented a Comprehensive Inventory Management System

VA's oversight of VAMC pharmacy inventory management is limited in part because VA currently lacks a comprehensive system that would allow the department and its VAMCs to monitor pharmacy inventory in real time. According to PBM officials, the lack of a VA-wide system makes it difficult to oversee VAMC pharmacy inventory management, and PBM has recognized the lack of such a system as a material weakness for several years. PBM officials said that implementation of a VA-wide pharmacy inventory management system would allow them to monitor each VAMC's pharmacy inventory in real time, which would, in turn, allow them to better manage inventory and help alleviate shortages at the national level by facilitating transfers of inventory between VAMCs as needed. Additionally, officials said that such a system would lead to better planning and projections for purchasing decisions, allow PBM to track medication expiration dates and lot numbers more effectively, and improve VAMC staff response to medication recalls.

Although VA has acknowledged the need for a VA-wide pharmacy inventory management system, such a system may not be available for the foreseeable future. PBM officials told us they have requested this system since the early 2000s. However, despite the documented technological challenges VA faces in overseeing its VAMC pharmacies, changing IT priorities, funding challenges, and the narrowing of the scope of a Pharmacy Re-engineering Project have prevented the system's development.[21] In 2017, we reported that VA's pharmacy systems could not maintain a real-time inventory across the VAMCs, and we recommended that VA assess the priority for establishing an inventory management system capable of monitoring medication inventory levels and indicating when medications needed to be reordered.[22] VA concurred with our recommendation. In June 2017, VA announced its intention to replace VistA— VA's health information system—with an off-the-shelf electronic health record system.[23] VA officials told us that the new system will have the capability to monitor pharmacy inventory in real time across VA. VA signed the contract for this new system in May 2018; however, full implementation is expected to take up to 10 years. In the interim, VA officials told us that while they will maintain current pharmacy systems,

[21] The Pharmacy Re-engineering Project began in 2002, and the original plans for this project included the development of inventory management capabilities. However, in June 2009 the Secretary of VA announced that VA would stop financing failed projects and improve the management of its IT development projects. Toward this end, the VA Chief Information Officer transitioned the Pharmacy Re-engineering Project to a phased development effort. According to VA pharmacy management officials, this was done because the project had faced funding delays, contracting difficulties, and differing directions from a number of VA chief information officers. The project was also re-scoped to focus on implementing clinical decision support tools, specifically to cross-check drugs in medication orders to reduce the frequency of adverse drug events and improve patient safety.

[22] GAO, *VA Information Technology: Pharmacy System Needs Additional Capabilities for Viewing, Exchanging, and Using Data to Better Serve Veterans*, GAO 17-179 (Washington, D.C.: June 14, 2017). In this report, we noted that industry practices stress the use of a computerized system to manage a real-time inventory so that the system displays up-to-date pharmaceutical inventory at all times. Interviews we conducted for this review with officials from the Mayo Clinic and the Cleveland Clinic—both large, integrated health systems similar to the VA—told us that they have systems in place that allow them to monitor medication levels in real time.

[23] The Department of Defense currently uses the same off-the-shelf electronic health record system, which is developed by Cerner. VA cited having all patient data residing in one common system and enabling seamless care between the Department of Veterans Affairs and the Department of Defense as a factor when choosing Cerner.

they do not plan to build any new systems—including a VA-wide pharmacy inventory management system—so they can efficiently manage resources in preparation for the transition to the new system.

VACO and VISNs Provide Some Limited Oversight, but VA Lacks a Focal Point for System-Wide Oversight of Pharmacy Inventory Management

	Entity	Responsibility
Headquarters level	Pharmacy Benefits Management Service (PBM)	• Develops policies for the provision of pharmacy services at the VAMCs. • Collects and aggregates data from VAMCs' pharmacy inventory on a quarterly and annual basis. • Facilitates regular calls with VISN and VAMC pharmacy staff to discuss pharmacy-related issues.
Headquarters level	National Acquisition Center (NAC)	• Coordinates with PBM on medication shortage issues and establishes national contracts for medications. • Administers the prime vendor contract.
Headquarters level	Office of Information and Technology (OIT)	• Develops computer systems based upon Veterans Health Administration prioritization and funding. • Assists VAMCs by troubleshooting issues that involve the Veterans Health Information Systems and Technology Architecture's pharmacy-related applications.
Regional level	Veterans Integrated Service Networks (VISN)	• Monitors data from quarterly and annual pharmacy inventories for VAMCs in their region.
Local level	VA medical centers (VAMC)	• Oversees VAMC pharmacy policies and the management of pharmacy inventory in accordance with VA policy.

Source: GAO analysis of VA documentation and interviews with officials. | GAO-18-658.

Figure 4. Department of Veterans Affairs' (VA) Entities That Have Pharmacy Inventory Management and Oversight Responsibilities.

VACO and the five VISNs we spoke with provide some limited oversight related to VAMC pharmacy inventory management, but no entity has system-wide responsibility for overseeing the performance of VAMC pharmacies in managing their inventories. Instead, responsibility for overseeing pharmacy inventory management is largely delegated to each VAMC's leadership. (See Figure 4 for a description of VACO headquarters, VISN, and VAMCs' roles and responsibilities in managing pharmacy inventory.)

PBM

In absence of a VA-wide inventory management system, PBM officials told us that they have employed manual workaround mechanisms to oversee pharmacy management processes. Specifically, PBM requires VAMC pharmacies to conduct an annual inventory of all medications and a quarterly inventory of 5 selected high-value non-controlled medications at risk of diversion.[24] PBM officials told us they remind VAMCs of the requirement to conduct these inventories, collect and aggregate the data from these inventories, and make summary reports from these data available as a resource to the VPEs and VAMC Chiefs of Pharmacy. PBM officials acknowledged that these manual workarounds are inefficient, increase labor costs, and leave the agency with an inability to see on-hand inventory across the system in real time. Additionally, the manual workarounds may be implemented differently at each VAMC, resulting in varying degrees of data reliability and limited opportunities for high-level oversight and data consolidation. PBM officials said that they do not independently analyze these data to identify trends, and they acknowledged that both the quarterly and annual inventories have limited usefulness for overseeing inventory management system-wide.[25] Additionally, officials at some of the selected VAMCs told us they found the quarterly and annual inventories to have limited usefulness for managing their pharmacy inventories.

---

[24] PBM instituted the requirement to conduct a quarterly inventory of 5 selected high-value, non-controlled substances at high risk of diversion in response to a 2009 VA OIG report that found that VA could not accurately account for the non-controlled medications at VAMC pharmacies because VA lacked reliable information to do so. See Department of Veterans Affairs, Office of Inspector General, *Audit of Veterans Health Administration's Management of Non-Controlled Drugs*, 08-01322-114 (Washington, D.C.: June 23, 2009).

[25] PBM officials told us they cannot conduct additional analyses on the self-reported data beyond calculating a high-level inventory turn rate at the VISN and VAMC level.

PBM officials told us they also hold regular meetings with VPEs and VAMCs, which provide the opportunity for discussion of pharmacy inventory management issues. However, our review of the minutes of the meetings between PBM and VPEs found that, over the past 3 years, pharmacy inventory management was rarely a topic of discussion. PBM officials noted that there is always an opportunity for open discussion at these meetings for VPEs to raise any issues, including issues related to pharmacy inventory management, but these discussions may or may not be captured in the meeting minutes.[26] PBM officials said they also regularly discuss various topics with the VAMC Chiefs of Pharmacy and other staff, but none of these calls are directly related to pharmacy inventory management.

NAC and OIT

Officials from VACO's NAC and OIT told us that they provide some assistance related to pharmacy inventory management but do not take part in the day-to-day management at the VAMC level and also do not have any oversight responsibilities. For example, a NAC official said the office coordinates with PBM on medication shortage issues and establishes national contracts for medications. NAC also sends out a weekly shortages report to various pharmacy groups as a tool to help them with known or expected shortages. Additionally, NAC's Pharmaceutical Prime Vendor team is responsible for administering the contract with the prime vendor through daily monitoring of issues and quarterly reviews with the prime vendor and PBM. OIT develops pharmacy-related applications for VistA based on requirements from PBM, and officials said that the majority of OIT's support to VAMCs consists of assisting them with issues related to VistA.[27]

---

[26] VA officials also noted that inventory management may also be discussed on conference calls and through email, but these discussions are not typically documented.

[27] Specifically, according to Veterans Health Administration officials, program offices such as PBM submit technology requests to the Office of Health Informatics for assessment. These requests are then submitted by the program offices to the Clinical Capabilities Management Board as part of their multi-year planning business plans. The Clinical Capabilities Management Board reviews these plans and provides input on the prioritization for

VISNs

At the VISN level, VPEs we interviewed also said they conduct some pharmacy inventory management oversight activities for the VAMCs within their network. While in general VA policy does not outline any specific roles for VPEs related to oversight of pharmacy inventory management, all five VPEs told us that they review the results of their VAMCs' annual inventories and discuss any issues that arise from this exercise with VAMCs as needed. VPEs told us that they also review the results of the quarterly inventory of five selected high-value, non-controlled substances and may follow-up with the VAMCs if their actual inventory of the medications is inconsistent with expected levels.[28] Additionally, some VPEs reported that they have undertaken additional oversight activities apart from reviewing results of the mandatory inventories. For example, one VPE told us he has developed a dashboard with 53 measures that, while focused on formulary management, also have inventory management implications. Additionally, this VPE said that a VISN-wide procurement work group meets on a monthly basis and serves as a venue for procurement technicians to share inventory management best practices. Such additional activities may be helpful, but since VPEs only have responsibility for VAMC pharmacies within their network, they may not be aware of pharmacy inventory management approaches being used at other VAMCs across VA.

Although VA offices at the headquarters and regional levels provide some assistance and oversight of how VAMCs manage pharmacy inventory at the local level, VA has not designated a focal point with defined responsibilities for system-wide oversight; instead they rely on local leadership to oversee pharmacy inventory management at the VAMCs. As a result, VA cannot assess the overall performance of VAMCs' management of their pharmacy inventories. The lack of a focal

technology requests, which are included in the Veterans Health Administration's budget request to OIT.

[28] VPEs we spoke with reported differing levels of acceptable variance between expected versus actual inventory for VAMCs' quarterly inventories of non-controlled substances. For example, one VPE said that the acceptable level of variance for VAMCs in his VISN should not be greater than 5 percent, while another VPE told us that the acceptable level of variance for VAMCs in her VISN is 10 percent.

point with defined oversight responsibilities is inconsistent with federal internal control standards for establishing structure and authority to achieve the entity's objectives and internal controls related to monitoring.[29] Specifically, internal controls state that management should establish an organizational structure, assign responsibility, and delegate authority to achieve the entity's objectives. Also, internal controls state that management should establish and operate monitoring activities to monitor the internal control system and evaluate the results. VA's actions are also inconsistent with the Office of Management and Budget's guidance for enterprise risk management and internal control in managing an agency.[30] Enterprise risk management is intended to yield an "enterprise-wide," strategically aligned portfolio view of organizational challenges that provides better insight about how to most effectively prioritize resource allocations to ensure successful mission delivery. Without a focal point for system-wide oversight of VAMC pharmacy inventory management, VA has limited awareness of the unique approaches that VAMCs use to manage their inventories and is missing an opportunity to evaluate these approaches. Additionally, VA cannot effectively share and standardize pharmacy inventory management best practices as appropriate. Having a focal point for system-wide oversight could allow VA to identify potential best practices that could be disseminated more widely across its facilities.

CONCLUSION

Due to the decentralized nature of VA's organization, VA policy gives VAMC pharmacies latitude in managing their pharmacy inventories.

---

[29] GAO-14-704G.

[30] Office of Management and Budget, *Management's Responsibility for Enterprise Risk Management and Internal Control*, Circular No. A-123 (July 15, 2016). Office of Management and Budget Circular No. A-123 prescribes requirements for conforming with the Standards of Internal Control in the Federal Government established by the Government Accountability Office, more commonly known as the Green Book. The guidance also specifies that agency management has responsibility for establishing and maintaining internal controls to achieve specific internal control objectives related to operations, reporting, and compliance. Lastly, the guidance discusses how internal control and enterprise risk management fit together to assist the agency in managing risks.

Several of the VAMCs we visited have taken unique approaches to procuring or tracking their inventory. However, because VA does not have a focal point to systematically oversee VAMCs' pharmacy management efforts, VA is missing opportunities to evaluate the effectiveness of these efforts, as well as share best practices and standardize them across VA as appropriate. PBM officials told us that the lack of a VA-wide pharmacy inventory management system limits their ability to oversee VAMC pharmacy inventory management. However, our review shows that even without this system there are existing mechanisms that a focal point could leverage to more systematically oversee how VAMC pharmacies manage their inventories. For example, a focal point could ensure that PBM officials, the VPEs, and VAMC pharmacy staff devote time to discussing pharmacy inventory management approaches and related issues during regularly scheduled telephone meetings. Leveraging these existing mechanisms is especially important given that VAMCs have historically had challenges in managing their inventories, and also because a VA-wide pharmacy inventory management system may not be available for the foreseeable future.

RECOMMENDATION FOR EXECUTIVE ACTION

We are making the following recommendation to the Department of Veterans Affairs:

The Secretary of the VA should direct the Undersecretary for Health to designate a focal point for overseeing VAMCs' pharmacy inventory management system-wide and define the focal point's responsibilities. (Recommendation 1)

AGENCY COMMENTS AND OUR EVALUATION

We provided a draft of this chapter to VA for review and comment. In its written comments, reproduced in appendix I, VA stated that it concurred in principle with our recommendation. VA also provided technical comments, which we incorporated as appropriate.

In response to our recommendation, VA stated it plans to establish by December 31, 2018, a committee of internal stakeholders and subject matter experts to provide options for overseeing VAMCs' pharmacy inventory management. However, it was unclear from VA's response whether the planned committee will recommend or designate an entity or focal point with system-wide oversight responsibilities. VA noted in its general comments that it does have entities or individuals—referred to as focal points by VA—responsible for specific functions. However, these entities do not provide system-wide oversight that could allow the department to better understand VAMCs' approaches to pharmacy inventory management. As we noted in our report, without a focal point for system-wide oversight, VA has limited awareness of the unique approaches that VAMCs use to manage their inventories and is missing an opportunity to evaluate these approaches and standardize them across VA as appropriate.

Additionally, in its general comments, VA raised concerns regarding our characterization in the draft report of medication shortages and the use of automated dispensing units in the context of controlled substances. In response, we updated the report to include more information about one VAMC's use of a committee to address medication shortages. We also clarified that three VAMCs are using (or will soon have the capability to use) enhanced analytic software to better leverage data generated through their automated dispensing machines, which allows them to more easily identify potential diversion. Finally, VA noted that we did not discuss PBM's multiple requests for an enterprise-management system since the early 2000s; however, this information was included as part of the draft report sent to VA for review and remains in our final report on page 14 as part of our finding on the lack of a VA-wide pharmacy inventory management system.

We are sending copies of this chapter to the Secretary of the Department of Veterans Affairs and appropriate congressional committees.

Sharon M. Silas
Acting Director, Health Care

APPENDIX I: COMMENTS FROM THE DEPARTMENT OF VETERANS AFFAIRS

THE SECRETARY OF VETERANS AFFAIRS
WASHINGTON
September 11, 2018

Ms. Sharon Silas
Acting Director
Health Care
U.S. Government Accountability Office
441 G Street, NW
Washington, DC 20548

Dear Ms. Silas:

The Department of Veterans Affairs (VA) has reviewed the Government Accountability Office (GAO) draft report: ***"VA HEALTH CARE: Pharmacy Inventory Management Could Benefit from System-Wide Oversight"*** (GAO-18-658).

The enclosure includes general and technical comments and sets forth the actions that will be taken to address the GAO draft report recommendation.

VA appreciates the opportunity to comment on your draft report.

Sincerely,

Robert L. Wilkie

Department of Veterans Affairs (VA) Comments to
Government Accountability Office (GAO) Draft Report
"VA HEALTH CARE: Pharmacy Inventory Management Could Benefit from System-Wide Oversight"
(GAO-18-658)

VA General Comments:

Throughout the draft report, GAO discusses medication shortages. We find that medication shortages are not caused by VA lacking an enterprise pharmacy inventory management system. Shortages have many causes and impact the entire United States health care system. Including medication shortages in the draft report could obscure the main issue, which is VA's long-standing lack of a pharmaceutical inventory system to track medications for accountability purposes. While we do not believe this report should include a discussion about medication shortages, if it does, there should be an explicit mention of supply chain disruptions that are unique to VA. Unlike VA, the private sector does not have restrictions through the Trade Agreements Act, the Buy American Act, or open market ordering inefficiencies. Some of the supply chain disruptions experienced by VA are legislative and regulatory in nature, and have nothing to do with inventory management deficiencies.

The Veterans Health Administration (VHA) Pharmacy Benefits Management (PBM) does not disagree that a shortage committee may be an effective resource. However, the opportunity to buy stock before it is no longer available, and when a shortage is known or expected, is generally a very tight window; and importantly, if VA hoards medications, other health care organizations will suffer. The committee would need to be extremely nimble to be effective at "preemptively mitigating shortages" should they occur, and PBM believes this is neither possible nor advisable.

VA agrees that inventory management includes procuring, receiving, storing, tracking, dispensing, and disposing of medications; however, it is only on page eleven that GAO notes that these functions are standardized and that there is a focal point for overseeing these activities: procuring (use of a national Pharmaceutical Prime Vendor based on VA National Contracts and Federal Supply Schedule contracts); receiving (separation of duties, internal control requirements); storing (policy requirements); dispensing (policy requirements); and disposing functions (VA National Contract). The major gap is that, because of a lack of an enterprise-wide system, VA has no reliable way to track medications from the time they are received until the time they are dispensed or destroyed. Some of that functionality is being performed through outpatient dispensing data; ward stock dispensing data; and inpatient drug distribution data. An exception to the lack of a tracking functionality is controlled substances, which are tracked from receipt through destruction. Tracking controlled substances through VA's Controlled Substance Tracking Package and automated dispensing units is the one area where VA has closed the gap in this process. What was attributed to two of the five medical centers is, in fact, required (use of the Controlled Substance Tracking package) or strongly recommended (use of automated dispensing cabinets).

VA General Comments:

Throughout the draft report, GAO discusses medication shortages. We find that medication shortages are not caused by VA lacking an enterprise pharmacy inventory management system. Shortages have many causes and impact the entire United States health care system. Including medication shortages in the draft report could obscure the main issue, which is VA's long-standing lack of a pharmaceutical inventory system to track medications for accountability purposes. While we do not believe this report should include a discussion about medication shortages, if it does, there should be an explicit mention of supply chain disruptions that are unique to VA. Unlike VA, the private sector does not have restrictions through the Trade Agreements Act, the Buy American Act, or open market ordering inefficiencies. Some of the supply chain disruptions experienced by VA are legislative and regulatory in nature, and have nothing to do with inventory management deficiencies.

The Veterans Health Administration (VHA) Pharmacy Benefits Management (PBM) does not disagree that a shortage committee may be an effective resource. However, the opportunity to buy stock before it is no longer available, and when a shortage is known or expected, is generally a very tight window; and importantly, if VA hoards medications, other health care organizations will suffer. The committee would need to be extremely nimble to be effective at "preemptively mitigating shortages" should they occur, and PBM believes this is neither possible nor advisable.

VA agrees that inventory management includes procuring, receiving, storing, tracking, dispensing, and disposing of medications; however, it is only on page eleven that GAO notes that these functions are standardized and that there is a focal point for overseeing these activities: procuring (use of a national Pharmaceutical Prime Vendor based on VA National Contracts and Federal Supply Schedule contracts); receiving (separation of duties, internal control requirements); storing (policy requirements); dispensing (policy requirements); and disposing functions (VA National Contract). The major gap is that, because of a lack of an enterprise-wide system, VA has no reliable way to track medications from the time they are received until the time they are dispensed or destroyed. Some of that functionality is being performed through outpatient dispensing data; ward stock dispensing data; and inpatient drug distribution data. An exception to the lack of a tracking functionality is controlled substances, which are tracked from receipt through destruction. Tracking controlled substances through VA's Controlled Substance Tracking Package and automated dispensing units is the one area where VA has closed the gap in this process. What was attributed to two of the five medical centers is, in fact, required (use of the Controlled Substance Tracking package) or strongly recommended (use of automated dispensing cabinets).

Additionally, the draft report fails to note that PBM has requested an enterprise-wide inventory management system since at least the early 2000s, well before numerous GAO and Office of Inspector General reviews were conducted on this topic. The lack of this type of system was not caused by PBM complacency or negligence, but rather because it has not been a development priority for VHA. The lack of this type of system also underscores and provides an important example of VA's failure to correct known system information technology deficiencies.

In June 2017, GAO published its final report ***"VA Information Technology: Pharmacy System Needs Additional Capabilities for Viewing, Exchanging, and Using Data to Better Serve Veterans"*** (GAO-17-179) including a recommendation to establish and implement a plan for updating the pharmacy inventory system to address the inefficiencies. The recommendation remains open at this time.

Recommendation 1: The Secretary of the VA should direct the Under Secretary for Health to designate a focal point for overseeing VAMCs' pharmacy inventory management system-wide and define the focal point's responsibilities.

VA Comments: Concur in principle. The Veterans Health Administration (VHA) agrees that a system-wide pharmacy inventory management system is critical to ensure the VA Central Office will address GAO's concerns. Therefore, VHA will establish a committee of internal stakeholders and subject matter experts to review GAO's recommendation and provide options to VHA's Executive in Charge for overseeing the VA medical centers' pharmacy inventory management systems. The status is in process with a target completion date of December 31, 2018.

In: Improvements Needed in the VA … ISBN: 978-1-53615-971-4
Editor: Charles Copeland

Chapter 10

VA HEALTH CARE: PROGRESS MADE TOWARDS IMPROVING OPIOID SAFETY, BUT FURTHER EFFORTS TO ASSESS PROGRESS AND REDUCE RISK ARE NEEDED*

United States Government Accountability Office

ABBREVIATIONS

CARA	Comprehensive Addiction and Recovery Act of 2016
DOD	Department of Defense
OSI	Opioid Safety Initiative
OTRR	Opioid Therapy Risk Report
PDMP	prescription drug monitoring program
STORM	Stratification Tool for Opioid Risk Mitigation
VA	Department of Veterans Affairs
VHA	Veterans Health Administration
VISN	Veterans Integrated Service Network.

* This is an edited, reformatted and augmented version of United States Government Accountability Office, Report to Congressional Committees, Publication No. GAO-18-380, dated May 2018.

Why GAO Did This Study

The Comprehensive Addiction and Recovery Act of 2016 and Senate Report 114-57 included provisions for GAO to report on VHA's OSI and the opioid prescribing practices of its health care providers.

This chapter examines, among other issues, (1) the extent to which VHA has met OSI goals established in 2014 and (2) the extent to which VHA providers adhere to key opioid risk mitigation strategies. To do this work, GAO reviewed data and documents related to OSI efforts and goals and interviewed VHA officials. In addition, GAO reviewed a random, nongeneralizable selection of medical records for 103 veterans who were prescribed opioids at five selected VHA medical facilities from March 2016 through March 2017. GAO selected the facilities to obtain diversity in geography and rates of opioid prescribing. At the selected facilities, GAO reviewed facility data and documents related to opioid safety and interviewed officials.

What GAO Recommends

GAO is making five recommendations to VHA, including that it document actions and develop measurable outcomes related to its OSI goals, ensure that providers are adhering to opioid risk mitigation strategies, and ensure that all its regional networks have implemented academic detailing programs and that all VHA medical facilities have a designated primary care pain champion, as required. The Department of Veterans Affairs concurred with GAO's recommendations and described steps it will take to implement them.

What GAO Found

The Veterans Health Administration (VHA) has made progress improving opioid safety through its Opioid Safety Initiative (OSI).

Launched in 2013, the OSI aims to help ensure that veterans are prescribed opioids in a safe and effective manner. Since the OSI began, VHA has seen reductions in opioid prescribing rates. For example, from the fourth quarter of fiscal year 2013 to the first quarter of fiscal year 2018, the percentage of patients dispensed an opioid decreased from about 17 percent to about 10 percent, or by about 267,000 veterans. Also, available evidence suggests VHA has accomplished six of nine OSI goals established in 2014; however, it is unclear whether the remaining three goals have been fully met. For example, in the case of OSI goal four (establishing safe and effective regional tapering programs for patients on opioids and benzodiazepines), GAO found that VHA lacked documentation that its regional networks established these programs. VHA also did not establish measures of safety or effectiveness under this goal. These limitations prevent VHA from fully evaluating progress and accurately determining the extent to which its efforts to help ensure safe and effective prescribing of opioids have been successful.

In a review of a nongeneralizable sample of 103 veterans' medical records at five selected VHA medical facilities, GAO found that VHA providers did not always adhere to key opioid risk mitigation strategies, which are required by VHA policy or relevant to OSI goals. For example, among 53 veterans who were prescribed long-term opioid therapy (defined as a 90-day supply in the last 6 months), GAO found that

- 40 veterans did not have their names queried in a state-run prescription drug monitoring program database. The databases are used to identify patients who are receiving multiple prescriptions that may place them at greater risk for misusing opioids or overdosing;
- 21 veterans did not have a urine drug screening within the year prior to having their prescription filled. The screenings are used to determine whether veterans are taking their opioid medications as prescribed; and
- 12 veterans did not provide written informed consent. Informed consent is a formal acknowledgement that the veteran has been

educated on the risks and benefits of opioid use prior to initiating long-term opioid therapy.

GAO found several factors that may have contributed to inconsistent adherence to key opioid risk mitigation strategies at the selected VHA facilities. For example, four of the five selected facilities did not have a pain champion (a primary care position required by VHA that can help providers adhere to opioid risk mitigation strategies), and not all facilities had access to academic detailing, a program in which trained clinical pharmacists work one-on-one with providers to better inform them about evidence-based care related to the appropriate treatment of relevant medical conditions. In addition, three of the five facilities did not consistently review veterans' medical records to ensure provider adherence to these strategies. To the extent that these factors affect all VHA facilities, VHA will continue to face challenges ensuring that its providers prescribe opioids in a safe and effective manner.

May 29, 2018
Congressional Committees

The United States is in the midst of an unprecedented opioid epidemic. According to 2016 data from the Substance and Mental Health Services Administration, nearly 12 million people age 12 or older misused opioids in the previous year. In addition, Centers for Disease Control data show that over 42,000 people died as a result of an opioid overdose in 2016—either from prescription opioids or illicit opioids such as heroin—a fivefold increase since 1999. According to the Department of Veterans Affairs' (VA) Veterans Health Administration (VHA), veterans are twice as likely to die from an accidental overdose when compared to the non-veteran population.

VHA has found that in its primary care settings, more than 50 percent of male veterans report having chronic pain, and the incidence among female veterans may be higher.[1] To help ensure that veterans are prescribed and use opioid pain medications in a safe and effective manner, VHA launched its national Opioid Safety Initiative (OSI) in 2013.[2] In 2014, VHA established a number of goals and requirements under the OSI aimed at improving the safety and care of veterans who are prescribed opioids for pain. In addition, in 2017, VA, along with the Department of Defense (DOD), updated its clinical practice guidelines related to opioid therapy for chronic pain to increase providers' awareness of evidence-based pain management practices.[3]

The Comprehensive Addiction and Recovery Act (CARA) of 2016 requires VA to implement a number of efforts aimed at improving opioid safety for veterans. CARA also includes a provision for GAO to assess VHA's recent efforts under the OSI as well as the opioid prescribing practices of VHA health care providers.[4] In addition, a Senate Report accompanying H.R. 2029, enacted as the 2016 Consolidated Appropriations Act, included a provision for GAO to review the effectiveness of the OSI and overall opioid prescribing patterns throughout VHA.[5] In this chapter, we

1. describe key efforts VHA has undertaken since 2013 as a part of the OSI;
2. examine the extent to which VHA has met its OSI goals established in 2014 and implemented certain provisions of CARA related to monitoring veterans who are prescribed opioids; and

---

[1] Veterans Affairs Academic Detailing Service, *Pain Management Opioid Safety VA Education Guide* (Washington, D.C.: 2014).

[2] According to VHA officials, the OSI rolled out nationwide during the 4th quarter of fiscal year 2013. Prior to the national roll out, according to officials, an OSI pilot task force was chartered in August 2012 and pilot programs were ongoing at various VHA facilities.

[3] Veterans Health Administration/Department of Defense, The Management of Opioid Therapy for Chronic Pain Working Group, *VA/DOD Clinical Practice Guideline for Management of Opioid Therapy for Chronic Pain* (Washington, D.C.: February 2017). Clinical practice guidelines are summaries of potential health care interventions designed to assist providers in their decision-making when creating a plan of care for a patient. Clinical practice guidelines typically describe the level of evidence associated with each intervention and provide recommendations based on that evidence.

[4] Comprehensive Addiction and Recovery Act of 2016, Pub. L. No. 114-198, § 913, 130 Stat. 695, 762.

[5] See Pub. L. No. 114-31,129 Stat. 2242 (2015); S. Rep. 114-57, at 47 (2015).

3. examine the extent to which VHA providers adhere to selected opioid risk mitigation strategies and clinical practice guideline recommendations related to prescribing opioids.

To describe key efforts VHA has undertaken since 2013 as a part of the OSI, we reviewed VHA documents and interviewed VHA Central Office officials regarding OSI efforts, including VHA efforts to monitor and address opioid prescribing patterns. We also analyzed data VHA collects under the OSI on four metrics related to rates of opioid prescribing and urine drug screening among certain veterans from the fourth quarter of fiscal year 2013 (roughly when the national OSI began at VHA) to the first quarter of fiscal year 2018, the most current quarter of data available at the time of our review. We also analyzed VHA data from its academic detailing programs on the frequency with which program representatives consulted with VHA providers on issues related to opioid safety.[6] We assessed the reliability of the data sources by reviewing relevant documentation, interviewing knowledgeable agency officials, and reviewing the data for missing values and outliers. Through these steps, we determined that the data were sufficiently reliable for the purposes of this reporting objective.

To examine VHA's progress on its 2014 OSI goals, we reviewed VHA documents and data relevant to OSI goals, including VHA opioid safety training data and OSI metric data. We also interviewed VHA Central Office officials, selected Veteran Integrated Service Network (VISN) officials, and VHA medical facility officials from 5 of 170 VHA medical facilities that we selected for our review.[7] We selected the 5 VHA medical facilities based on variation in geography and to reflect the full range of variation in the rate of change over time in the percentage of veterans who

[6] Academic detailing is a program in which trained clinical pharmacists work one-on-one with providers to better inform them about evidence-based care related to the appropriate treatment of relevant medical conditions.

[7] VISNs are regional networks that manage the VHA medical facilities located in their region. In October 2015, VHA began to implement a realignment of its VISN boundaries which will result in the number of its VISNs decreasing from 21 to 18. For the purposes of this report, "VHA medical facilities" refers to medical centers, health care systems, or outpatient centers, including any affiliated community-based clinics.

have been prescribed an opioid.[8] Our findings from the selected facilities are not generalizable to all VHA medical facilities. We examined VHA's progress on its OSI goals in the context of federal internal control standards for documentation requirements and the establishment and review of performance measures and indicators.[9] We assessed the reliability of the data sources by reviewing relevant documentation, interviewing knowledgeable agency officials, and reviewing the data for missing values and outliers. Through these steps, for the purposes of this reporting objective, we determined that the VISN-level opioid safety training assignment data were not reliable; however, all other data sources we analyzed were sufficiently reliable. To assess whether VHA is meeting certain provisions of CARA related to monitoring veterans who are prescribed opioids, we interviewed VHA Central Office officials and reviewed documents related to these provisions.[10]

To examine the extent to which VHA providers adhere to selected opioid risk mitigation strategies and clinical practice guideline recommendations related to prescription opioid therapy, we focused on three key VHA opioid risk mitigation strategies and three VA/DOD

---

[8] Based on the OSI metric represented by the percentage of patients dispensed an opioid, we calculated the change over time from quarter 4, fiscal year 2012 through quarter 1, fiscal year 2017 for all VHA facilities, including the average change over time of all facilities. We selected one facility that exhibited the average change, two facilities above the average change, and two facilities below the average change. All facilities experienced a decrease in this metric over this time period except one, which experienced no change, while one facility in Manila, Philippines experienced an increase. Our selection process resulted in one facility that had among the greatest decreases and one facility that had among the lowest decreases. The VHA medical facilities we included in our review are based in Roseburg, OR (VISN 20); Hampton, VA (VISN 6); Columbus, OH (VISN 10); Tuscaloosa, AL (VISN 7); and Minneapolis, MN (VISN 23).

[9] GAO, *Standards for Internal Control in the Federal Government*, GAO-14-704G (Washington, D.C.: Sept. 10, 2014) and *Standards for Internal Control in the Federal Government*, GAO/AIMD-00-21.3.1 (Washington, D.C.: Nov. 1, 1999). Internal control is a process effected by an entity's management, oversight body, and other personnel that provides reasonable assurance that the objectives of an entity will be achieved.

[10] CARA requires VHA to ensure that the Opioid Therapy Risk Report (OTRR), an opioid safety monitoring tool, has the ability to track whether a provider prescribed opioids to a veteran without first checking the information in the tool and to include in the OTRR information on the most recent time the tool was accessed by a provider. In addition, CARA requires VHA to modify its electronic medical record system to notify providers if a veteran is receiving opioid therapy and has a history of substance use disorder or prior overdose; has a history of opioid abuse; or is at risk of developing an opioid use disorder.

clinical practice guideline recommendations—all of which, generally speaking, are strong evidence-based strategies for reducing the potential health risks associated with opioid use.[11] The three opioid risk mitigation strategies are the following:

- an annual urine drug screening for patients on long-term opioid therapy (defined by VHA as having had a 90-day supply in the last 6 months; increasing these screenings is an explicit goal of the OSI;
- a VHA-required annual query of a prescription database maintained by a state prescription drug monitoring program when prescribing controlled substances, including opioids, to check for whether patients are receiving multiple prescriptions;[12] and
- obtaining written informed consent from patients on the use of opioids so that they have an informed understanding of the medications' risks and benefits, as required by VHA policy.[13]

The three clinical practice guideline recommendations are the following:

- the use of non-pharmacological treatments (such as cognitive behavioral therapy and yoga) in addition to or in lieu of opioid therapy;
- the prescribing of naloxone to help reverse opioid overdoses; and
- appropriate follow-up visits with a provider after an opioid is prescribed and after an opioid prescription is changed.[14]

---

[11] *VA/DOD Clinical Practice Guideline for Management of Opioid Therapy for Chronic Pain.* The guideline contains 18 recommendations.

[12] Veterans Health Administration, *Querying State Prescription Drug Monitoring Programs*, VHA Directive 1306 (Washington, D.C.: Oct.19, 2016). This requirement is subject to limitations imposed by states on VA's access to state prescription drug monitoring databases.

[13] Veterans Health Administration, *Informed Consent for Long-Term Opioid Therapy for Pain*, VHA Directive 1005 (Washington, D.C.: May 6, 2014). This requirement does not apply to patients enrolled in hospice or patients receiving long-term opioids for cancer pain.

[14] Guidance on the appropriate timing of pain management follow-up visits is provided in both the 2017 and 2010 VA/DOD clinical practice guidelines. Under the 2017 recommendation,

To assess adherence to these opioid risk mitigation strategies and guideline recommendations, we reviewed a random, nongeneralizable sample of medical records for 103 veterans who had received long-term opioid therapy between March 1, 2016 and March 31, 2017. The 103 records we reviewed included a minimum of 20 records each from our five selected facilities. The sample of records also included records for 50 veterans at a greater risk of adverse events due to opioid use, including 25 veterans who received benzodiazepines concurrently with an opioid and another 25 veterans who were categorized as "very high" risk in VHA's opioid safety monitoring tool, the Stratification Tool for Opioid Risk Mitigation (STORM), during the summer and fall of 2017 when the medical record review was conducted.[15] As part of our work, we also reviewed relevant documents and interviewed officials from the five selected VHA medical facilities, the VISNs associated with the facilities, and VHA Central Office.

We conducted this performance audit from November 2016 to May 2018 in accordance with generally accepted government auditing standards. Those standards require that we plan and perform the audit to obtain sufficient, appropriate evidence to provide a reasonable basis for our findings and conclusions based on our audit objectives. We believe that the evidence obtained provides a reasonable basis for our findings and conclusions based on our audit objectives.

---

follow-up pain management visits should be scheduled at least every 1- 4 weeks after any change in medication regimen and at least once every 1-3 months for the duration of the therapy. This was a change from the 2010 recommendation, which we used for our analysis. The 2010 recommendation states that follow-up visits should be scheduled at least every 2-4 weeks after any change in medication regimen and at least once every 1-6 months for the duration of the therapy.

[15] Benzodiazepines are a type of depressant that, among other things, produces sedation and relieves anxiety (e.g., Valium and Xanax). According to the 2017 VA/DOD clinical practice guideline for chronic pain, there is evidence that using opioids and benzodiazepines concurrently increases the risk of overdose and overdose death and therefore is not recommended. STORM is a clinical tool that provides 1-year and 3-year risk categories (i.e., low, medium, high, and very high) reflecting a patient's risk of an adverse event if opioids are prescribed, based on the veteran's individual medical history and characteristics. The 25 veterans we reviewed had "very high" risk categories for both the 1-year and 3-year estimates. For example, a patient with an 18 percent risk of a suicide- or overdose-related health care event or death in the next year would be categorized as "very high" risk by the tool.

BACKGROUND

OSI Goals and Related Requirements

Table 1. Veterans Health Administration (VHA) Opioid Safety Initiative (OSI) goals and required actions, December 2014

OSI goal	VHA-required action
(1) Educate opioid prescribers regarding the effective use of urine drug screening	Veteran Integrated Service Networks (VISN) will establish a network-wide standardized education program by December 31, 2014
(2) Increase the use of urine drug screening	Urine drug screening targets based on previous urine drug screening rates for all VHA facilities by quarter 2, fiscal year 2015
(3) Facilitate the use of prescription drug monitoring program databases containing patient-level information on prescriptions for controlled substances	VISNs must certify by quarter 2, fiscal year 2015 that facilities have an education program that consists of training and/or education materials for providers
(4) Establish safe and effective VISN tapering programs for veterans using opioids and benzodiazepines	VISNs must develop local tapering protocols and plans to resource the implementation of those tapering protocols
(5) Develop tools to identify veterans at a higher risk for adverse events while using opioids	Develop an opioid risk stratification toolkit; opioid safety education guides must be updated annually
(6) Improve prescribing practices around long-acting opioid formulations	VISNs need to develop local tapering protocols and plans to resource the implementation of those tapering protocols
(7) Review treatment plans for veterans on high doses of opioids	VISN certification that patients with greater than a 200 morphine milligram equivalent dose per day have been reviewed by quarter 2, fiscal year 2015
(8) Offer complementary and alternative medicine modalities for chronic pain at all medical facilities	Each facility must provide evidence that at least two evidence-based behavioral/psychological treatments or approved complementary or alternative modalities can be provided by quarter 2, fiscal year 2015[a]
(9) Develop new models of mental health and primary care collaboration to manage the prescribing of opioids and benzodiazepines in patients with chronic pain	Identify strong practices that can be operationalized across VHA by quarter 3, fiscal year 2015; a request for proposal to be released to the field to establish model interdisciplinary teams and strategies for management and tapering of medications at three VHA medical facilities

Source: VHA. | GAO-18-380.

[a]According to VHA, evidence-based behavioral/psychological treatments include cognitive behavioral therapy for pain and relaxation practices, and approved complementary and alternative modalities include acupuncture, acupressure, yoga and progressive relaxation.

To help ensure that veterans are prescribed and use opioid pain medications in a safe and effective manner, VHA launched its OSI nationally in 2013. VHA established nine OSI goals in a December 2014 memorandum. For each of the goals, VHA directed its VISNs and their associated VHA medical facilities to take specified actions to meet the goals (See Table 1).

VHA has also developed opioid risk mitigation strategies for its providers to follow when prescribing opioid pain medications to veterans. These key strategies include one whose increased use is an explicit goal for the OSI and two that are requirements in VHA policy.

1. Annual urine drug screening for veterans on long-term opioid therapy. Providers should generally ensure that a urine drug screening has been conducted for veterans who are on long-term opioid therapy at least once in the 365 days prior to initiating or renewing an opioid prescription.[17] Urine drug screening allows providers to monitor the types of drugs that are in a veteran's system, including controlled and illicit substances. Increasing the use of urine drug screening is OSI goal two.
2. Annual prescription drug monitoring program (PDMP) query. PDMPs are state-run electronic databases used to track the prescribing and dispensing of prescriptions for controlled substances, identify suspected misuse or diversion (i.e., channeling drugs into illegal use), and identify trends in drug utilization. In 2016, VHA began requiring in policy that providers query state PDMPs at least once annually when prescribing opioids to determine whether their patients have received prescriptions for opioid medications or other controlled substances from non-VA providers.[18]

---

[17] VHA defines long-term opioid therapy as having had a 90-day supply or more of opioids in the last 6 months.

[18] Veterans Health Administration, *Querying State Prescription Drug Monitoring Programs*, VHA Directive 1306 (Washington, D.C.: Oct.19, 2016). This requirement is subject to limitations imposed by states, which can impact VHA providers' access to PDMP databases. According to VHA policy, providers should follow state regulations for PDMP queries if these regulations are more stringent than VHA's policy.

3. Informed consent for long-term opioid therapy. In 2014, VHA began requiring in policy that providers educate their patients on the risks associated with the use of prescription opioids and to obtain veterans' formal acknowledgment of these risks in writing prior to initiating longterm opioid therapy.[19]

Clinical Practice Guidelines for the Treatment of Chronic Pain

In 2010, in coordination with DOD, VA developed clinical practice guidelines for its providers to use when prescribing opioids for chronic pain. These guidelines were updated in 2017.[20] While clinical practice guidelines contain evidence-based recommendations, they are not required to be followed in all clinical situations; therefore, variations in practice may occur based on individual patient needs subject to the discretion of the provider.

The 2017 VA/DOD clinical practice guidelines related to opioid therapy for chronic pain generally complement VHA's OSI goals. For example, the guidelines recommend a conservative use of opioids for chronic pain and emphasize strategies to mitigate the risk of using opioids. The evidence-based clinical practice guideline recommendations include the following:

1. Use of non-pharmacological treatments. The guidelines advise not initiating opioid therapy for chronic pain. They also recommend alternatives to opioid therapy, such as non-opioid medications and non-pharmacological treatments. Non-pharmacological treatments

---

[19] Veterans Health Administration, *Informed Consent for Long-Term Opioid Therapy for Pain*, VHA Directive 1005 (Washington, D.C.: May 6, 2014). This requirement does not apply to patients enrolled in hospice or patients receiving long-term opioids for cancer pain.

[20] A Senate report directed VA, in consultation with DOD, to update its clinical practice guideline for chronic pain no later than December 31, 2016. See S. Rep. No. 114-57, at 46 (2015). According to a VHA official, generally speaking, the recommendations contained in the VA/DOD clinical practice guideline for opioid therapy for chronic pain are largely consistent with the Centers for Disease Control's 2016 Guideline for Prescribing Opioids for Chronic Pain. See Centers for Disease Control, *CDC Guideline for Prescribing Opioids for Chronic Pain – United States, 2016* (Atlanta: March 18, 2016).

for chronic pain include, for example, cognitive behavioral therapy and yoga.

2. Naloxone prescribing. Naloxone is a highly effective, potentially lifesaving intervention for reversing opioid overdoses, and it can be prescribed to veterans as a preventive measure. Veterans who are prescribed naloxone can use it when experiencing an overdose or a family member can administer it on their behalf. According to the clinical practice guidelines, naloxone should be offered as an antidote to all patients at risk for an opioid overdose, including those who are in the process of tapering from opioids.[21] The guidelines describe several significant risk factors which can indicate the prescribing of naloxone, including the duration and dose of opioids, current or history of depression or substance use disorder, and suicidality.
3. Appropriate follow-up visits with a provider. According to the guidelines, follow-up pain management visits should be scheduled at least every 1-4 weeks after any change in medication regimen and at least once every 1-3 months for the duration of the therapy to help ensure that the treatment plan is optimized.[22]

UNDER ITS OSI, VHA TRACKS OPIOID PRESCRIBING PATTERNS, IDENTIFIES PRESCRIBING OUTLIERS, AND EDUCATES PRESCRIBERS

VHA officials told us that the main focus of the OSI is changing the prescribing patterns of providers to better align with evidence-based practices. We found that this has been carried out by VHA through three

---

[21] CARA directs VHA to maximize the availability of naloxone to veterans and to ensure that veterans who are considered at risk for opioid overdose have access to naloxone and training on its proper administration. Comprehensive Addiction and Recovery Act of 2016, Pub. L. No. 114-198, § 911(e)(1), 130 Stat. 695, 759.

[22] This 2017 recommendation represents a change from the 2010 clinical practice guideline, which states that follow-up visits should be scheduled at least every 1-4 weeks after any change in medication regimen and at least once every 1-6 months for the duration of the therapy.

key efforts: tracking opioid prescribing rates and other trends, identifying irregular prescribing patterns, and educating providers on best practices through academic detailing.

Tracking Opioid Prescribing Patterns

Under the OSI, VHA uses quarterly data derived from VHA's electronic medical record system to monitor prescription opioid use among veterans, the related prescribing patterns of VHA providers, and the rates of urine drug screening for veterans receiving long-term opioid therapy.[23] Specifically, VHA tracks the following four clinical indicators, known as the OSI metrics, for each of its medical facilities:

1. the percentage of patients dispensed an opioid,
2. the percentage of patients dispensed an opioid and a benzodiazepine,
3. the percentage of patients on long-term opioid therapy who received a urine drug screen within the previous year of having their prescription filled, and
4. the percentage of patients dispensed greater than or equal to 100 morphine milligram equivalents per day.[24]

Our analysis of quarterly OSI metric data shows that since the beginning of the OSI in the fourth quarter of fiscal year 2013 to the first quarter of fiscal year 2018 (the most recent data available at the time of our review), the percentage of veterans dispensed an opioid has decreased by 7 percentage points, or roughly 267,000 veterans, while the rate of urine drug

[23] VHA defines long-term opioid therapy as having had a 90-day supply or more of opioids in the last 6 months. VHA began making the quarterly opioid prescribing data it tracks publicly available in January 2018. See https://www.data.va.gov/story/department-veterans-affairs-opioid-prescribing-data (last access date: March 14, 2018).

[24] The 2017 VA/DOD clinical practice guideline for chronic pain does not recommend opioid doses of greater than 90 morphine milligram equivalents per day

screening for veterans on long-term opioid therapy increased significantly—by over 47 percentage points.

Table 2. Changes in Veterans Health Administration (VHA) Opioid Safety Initiative (OSI) metrics, Fourth Quarter Fiscal Year 2014 through First Quarter, Fiscal Year 2018

OSI metric	Fiscal year 2013 (4th quarter)	Fiscal year 2018 (1st quarter)	Percentage point change
Percentage of patients dispensed an opioid[a]	16.7 (665,786 of 3,984,165 patients)	9.7 (398,899 of 4,130,536 patients)	- 7.1 (- 266,887 patients)
Percentage of patients dispensed an opioid and a benzodiazepine[b]	13.2 (116,739 / 885,142)	6.6 (36,938 / 558,199)	- 6.6 (- 79,801)
Percentage of patients on long term opioid therapy having received a urine drug screen within the previous year of having their prescription filled[c]	42.2 (182,194 / 431,694)	89.2 (209,102 / 234,392)	+ 47.0e (+ 26,908)
Percentage of patients dispensed greater than or equal to a 100 morphine milligram equivalents per day[d]	6.5 (56,831 / 869,956)	4.4 (23,968 / 543,782)	- 2.1 (- 32,863)

Source: VHA. | GAO-18-380. Notes: 4th quarter, fiscal year 2013=July to September 2013. 1st quarter, fiscal year 2018=October to December 2017.

[a]Denominator=patients who were dispensed at least one outpatient prescription during the reporting timeframe.

[b]Denominator=patients who were dispensed opioids, including tramadol, in the reporting timeframe.

[c]Denominator=patients who were dispensed at least one opioid medication in the reporting timeframe and had a total supply of opioids greater than or equal to 90 days for the selected quarter and the prior quarter. Increasing the use of urine drug screening is an explicit goal of the OSI.

[d]Denominator=patients who were dispensed opioids, including tramadol, in the reporting timeframe. The 2017 VA/DOD clinical practice guideline for chronic pain does not recommend opioid doses of greater than 90 morphine milligram equivalents per day.

[e]The increase in the rate of urine drug screening was driven more by a reduction in the number of veterans on long-term opioid therapy than an increase in the number of veterans receiving screening over time.

The increase in the percentage of patients receiving a urine drug screening was driven more by a reduction in the total number of patients on long-term opioid therapy (about 197,000 veterans) than an increase in the number of patients receiving the screening (about 27,000 veterans) (See Table 2).

Identifying Irregular Prescribing Patterns

As part of its monitoring of the OSI metrics, VHA Central Office has periodically identified VHA medical facilities and VHA providers who deviate from average prescribing rates across VHA. For example:

- *Facilities.* In 2014, VHA Central Office identified 39 of 140 medical facilities across 12 VISNs with relatively higher rates of opioid dispensing as outliers based on the OSI metric percentage of veterans dispensed an opioid.[25] VHA Central Office notified the VISNs of these facilities and required each facility to submit a corrective action plan to VHA Central Office outlining the actions they would take to reduce opioid prescribing. Based on our analysis of VHA documents, we found that the identified facilities in the five VISNs selected for our review submitted information in response to VHA Central Office's request.[26]
- *Providers.* In February 2017, VHA Central Office identified 320 outliers out of 8,351 providers at 94 VHA medical facilities based on the relatively high proportion of their patients who were prescribed opioids.[27] VHA Central Office directed the VHA medical facilities associated with these outlier providers to review their prescribing rates in the context of their clinical practice, and to report back with any feedback given or actions taken. According to officials from the five facilities in our review, outlier providers tended to be surgeons, pain management specialists, or physical rehabilitation providers who might be expected to prescribe

[25] Outlier VHA medical facilities were flagged if the facility's rate of decrease in opioid dispensing between fiscal year 2012 to fiscal year 2014 was less than the national rate of decrease, or if opioid dispensing increased during this time period.

[26] We did not review the extent to which these VHA medical facilities completed the steps identified in their action plan or the extent to which VISNs or VHA Central Office monitored the completion of the action plans.

[27] Providers were identified as outliers if (1) the provider wrote at least one opioid prescription; (2) prescribed at least one medication of any type to a minimum of 150 veterans from October 2016 through December 2016; and (3) the provider's percentage of opioid prescriptions was greater than two standard deviations from the national mean for the same time period.

opioids at a higher-than-average rate due to the nature of their specialty and the types of patients they treat. According to a VHA Central Office progress report, the facilities provided feedback and follow-up actions for 319 out of 320 outlier providers.[28] In May 2017, VHA identified a second round of 303 outliers out of 8,505 providers; 187 of these providers were previously identified as outliers in February 2017.[29] According to one VHA Central Office official, as of September 2017, VHA was reviewing these outlier data and will evaluate whether VHA facilities will be asked to conduct further reviews of these prescribers.

Educating Providers through Academic Detailing

To help change the prescribing patterns of providers, VHA has also implemented a system-wide academic detailing program to educate providers and improve the delivery of evidence-based health care at facilities. In 2015, VHA required each VISN to establish such a program to improve performance on all OSI metrics.[30] According to VHA Central Office officials, academic detailers are responsible for reviewing facility-level data on the prescribing patterns of providers and identifying potential areas of improvement. Detailers can educate providers with higher-than-average prescribing rates—such as those outliers identified in February and May 2017 by VHA Central Office—to help ensure providers are delivering safe and effective care for pain.

According to VHA, as of January 2018, academic detailers have conducted over 20,000 opioid-related visits to VHA providers. According to VHA officials, their data also show that academic detailing results in greater patient safety for veterans taking opioids. For example, compared

[28] While we discussed these responses with facility officials in our review, we did not verify or evaluate any actions taken in response to outlier prescribers.

[29] Providers were identified as outliers if (1) the provider wrote at least one opioid prescription; (2) prescribed at least one medication of any type to a minimum of 150 veterans from January 2017 through March 2017; and (3) the provider's percentage of opioid prescriptions was greater than two standard deviations from the national mean for the same time period.

[30] VHA Central Office requires a minimum of three full-time equivalent detailers for each VISN.

with those who did not receive academic detailing visits, providers who did receive such visits experienced (1) greater reductions in the proportion of their patients on high-dose opioids, (2) reductions in their patients' average morphine milligram equivalent daily dosage, and (3) increases in their naloxone prescribing rates.[31]

VHA Has Made Progress on OSI Goals, But Performance Measurement Limitations Exist for Some Goals and Certain CARA Provisions Have Not Been Fully Implemented

VHA Has Made Progress on Many 2014 OSI Goals, but for Some Goals, Performance Measurement Limitations Prevent an Accurate Determination of their Completion

Based on our analysis of VHA information, we found evidence suggesting that the agency has accomplished six of the nine 2014 OSI goals. For example, the agency has seen increases in the use of urine drug screening for veterans on long-term opioid therapy, and it has developed provider tools to identify veterans at a higher risk for adverse events while using opioids. For several goals, although VHA did not implement the actions required in all those instances, the agency provided us with information or data demonstrating that the goals had effectively been met.

[31] For example, according to VHA, their data show that from October 2013 to September 2016, the proportion of patients on high-dose opioids decreased by 58 percent among providers who had received an academic detailing visit, compared to a 34 percent decrease among providers who did not receive an academic detailing visit. From October 2015 to September 2016, the average morphine milligram equivalent daily dosage decreased 59 percent among providers who met with a detailer, compared to 31 percent for those who did not. Finally, 1 year after visiting with a detailer, the average number of naloxone prescriptions per month was three times greater among providers who received an academic detailing visit compared with those who did not. See M Bounthavong et al. "Trends in naloxone prescriptions prescribed after implementation of a National Academic Detailing Service in the Veterans Health Administration: A preliminary analysis." *Journal of the American Pharmacists Association* (2017) S68-S72.

Table 3. Status of Veterans Health Administration (VHA) 2014 Opioid Safety Initiative (OSI) Goals as of March 2018

Goals	VHA required action(s)	Were these required action(s) completed?	Did VHA provide documentation that other actions met the goal?
(1) Educate opioid prescribers regarding the effective use of urine drug screening	Each VISN must establish a network-wide standardized education program by December 31, 2014	No	Yes
(2) Increase the use of urine drug screening	Urine drug screening targets based on previous urine drug screening rates for all VHA facilities must be reached by quarter 2, fiscal year 2015 (March 31, 2015)	No	Yes
(3) Facilitate the use of prescription drug monitoring program (PDMP) databases, which contain patient-level information on prescriptions received for controlled substances	Each VISN must certify by quarter 2, fiscal year 2015 (March 31, 2015), that all facilities have a program consisting of PDMP training and/or education materials for providers	No	Yes
(4) Establish safe and effective Veteran Integrated Service Network (VISN) tapering programs for veterans using opioids and benzodiazepines	VISNs must develop local tapering protocols and plans to resource the implementation of those tapering protocols	No	No. VHA lacks documentation related to the required action and could not provide evidence to indicate the goal was accomplished.
(5) Develop tools to identify veterans at a higher risk for adverse events while using opioids	An opioid risk stratification toolkit must be developed; opioid safety education guides must be updated annually	Yes	Yes
(6) Improve prescribing practices around long-acting opioid formulations	VISNs must develop local tapering protocols and plans to resource the implementation of those tapering protocols	No	Yes
(7) Review treatment plans for veterans on high doses of opioids	Each VISN must certify that the treatment of all patients with greater than a 200 morphine milligram equivalent dose per day has been reviewed by quarter 2, fiscal year 2015 (March 31, 2015)	No	No. VHA lacks documentation related to the required action and could not provide evidence to indicate

Table 3. (Continued)

Goals	VHA required action(s)	Were these required action(s) completed?	Did VHA provide documentation that other actions met the goal?
			the goal was accomplished.
(8) Offer complementary and alternative medicine modalities for chronic pain at all medical facilities	Each facility must provide evidence that at least one evidence-based psychosocial service and one approved complementary and integrative service is available by quarter 2, fiscal year 2015 (March 31, 2015)	Yes	Yes
(9) Develop new models of mental health and primary care collaboration to manage the prescribing of opioids and benzodiazepines in patients with chronic pain	Identify strong practices that can be operationalized across VHA by quarter 3, fiscal year 2015 (June 30, 2015); a request for proposal to be released to the field to establish model interdisciplinary teams and strategies for management and tapering of medications at three VHA medical facilities	No	To be determined. VHA reported other actions are underway to address this goal.

Source: GAO analysis of VHA information. | GAO-18-380.

However, for three OSI goals, it is unclear if the goal has been fully met because VHA lacks documentation showing that it has implemented the required action under the goal or the required action is still in progress. (See Table 3). (See appendix I for a more detailed description of VHA's known efforts and data related to each goal).

When asked about the lack of documentation for two of its OSI goals (goals four and seven), VHA officials told us that relevant documentation could not be produced. This lack of documentation is inconsistent with federal internal control standards. Specifically, according to federal internal control standards, management should evaluate and document the results of monitoring.[33] By not documenting the actions it is taking under each of its OSI goals, VHA lacks assurance that these actions have been

[33] GAO-14-704G and GAO/AIMD-00-21.3.1.

implemented by the VISNs or VHA medical facilities. As a result, VHA does not know whether it has fully met these OSI goals.

Moreover, for the OSI goal related to establishing safe and effective VISN tapering programs for veterans using opioids and benzodiazepines (goal four), VHA officials told us that they addressed this goal by issuing national tapering guidance, including a provider reference guide in 2014, an opioid taper decision tool in 2016, and the VA/DOD clinical practice guidelines in 2017. However, these actions do not appear to be sufficient for meeting the goal as it is currently written, because issuing national guidance alone does not ensure that safe and effective tapering programs are established.[34] Furthermore, VHA did not specify how safety and effectiveness within a tapering program would be measured, nor did the agency specify a deadline for the required action as described in December 2014. According to federal internal control standards relating to the establishment and review of performance measures and indicators, government agencies should use appropriate information to adequately assess performance, including establishing milestones or numerical targets, as appropriate.[35] Without clearly defined and measurable outcomes, VHA cannot fully assess its progress towards meeting this OSI goal.

VHA Has Not Implemented Certain CARA Requirements Related to Monitoring Veterans Prescribed Opioids

We also found that VHA has not implemented two CARA requirements intended to improve opioid safety for veterans.

---

[34] VHA officials told us they have not updated the 2014 OSI goals since the December 2014 memo was issued. According to one VHA official, CARA requirements and the issuance of the VA/DOD clinical practice guideline for chronic pain superseded the 2014 OSI goals and made any follow-up of the 2014 OSI goals obsolete. However, VHA did not provide any documentation during our review indicating that VHA Central Office determined that the 2014 OSI goals became obsolete given new priorities or that this determination was communicated to the medical facilities.

[35] GAO-14-704G and GAO/AIMD-00-21.3.1.

First, CARA requires that VHA's Opioid Therapy Risk Report (OTRR) have the ability to determine whether a provider has prescribed opioids to a veteran without checking that veteran's information in the OTRR.[36] Available to providers through VHA's electronic medical record system, OTRR is a clinical tool that provides information on any opioid and concurrent benzodiazepine prescriptions a veteran is receiving, the veteran's current and prior health conditions, recent and upcoming appointments, and whether any opioid risk mitigation strategies have been employed (such as urine drug screening or PDMP query).[37] However, we found that VHA Central Office cannot track the extent to which VHA providers use OTRR because this tool does not have this tracking capability.[38] VHA officials said that adding tracking capabilities to OTRR is not a high priority for the agency due to limited resources and competing priorities. Instead, according to a draft memorandum, VHA Central Office is planning to address this CARA provision by requiring VHA providers to document the use of OTRR in a standardized way that VHA can monitor. However, as of March 2018, VHA has not established this requirement or outlined the process for monitoring providers' use of OTRR.

---

[36] CARA requires the Secretary to include in the OTRR tool information on the most recent time the tool was accessed by a provider with respect to each veteran as well as information on the results of the most recent urine drug test for each veteran. See Pub. L. No. 114-198, § 911(f), 130 Stat. 695, 759. CARA also states that the Secretary shall establish guidance that each provider, before initiating opioid therapy to treat a patient as part of the comprehensive assessment conducted by the health care provider, use the OTRR tool (or any subsequent tool). Pub. L. No. 114-198, § 911(a)(2), 130 Stat. 695, 756.

[37] VHA has another tool, STORM, available to providers to help monitor patients prescribed opioids. It provides risk scores based on veterans' individual medical histories and characteristics indicating the risk of an adverse event if opioids are prescribed. To help providers determine the level of risk if an opioid prescription is started, increased, or reduced, hypothetical risk scores are available to providers through STORM. According to VHA officials, the agency plans to meet some CARA requirements with STORM rather than OTRR.

[38] VHA is able to track generally how many times providers have accessed OTRR, but OTRR cannot provide any more specific details, such as which providers accessed the tool and whether they did so prior to initiating opioid therapy for a particular veteran. In the case of STORM, officials said that they can tell whether providers have accessed STORM, but they cannot track which particular veterans were reviewed.

Without the ability to track the use of OTRR, VHA cannot sufficiently monitor whether providers are using the tool to help reduce the likelihood of opioid-related adverse events occurring among veterans receiving care through VHA.

CARA also requires that VHA modify its electronic medical record system so that any provider who accesses the record of a veteran will be notified whether that veteran is receiving opioid therapy and has a history of substance abuse disorder or prior instances of overdose; has a history of opioid abuse; or is at risk of developing an opioid use disorder. However, we found that VHA does not plan to modify its electronic medical record system to implement this capability. When asked about this provision in CARA, VHA officials said that VHA's medical record currently has real-time alerts to inform providers about veterans' existing opioid prescriptions and that any patient exposed to an opioid could be at risk of developing an opioid use disorder. Additionally, they said that an alert regarding current or past history of opioid use disorder could have an unintended consequence of discouraging veterans from reporting their medical history due to the stigma surrounding drug use disorders.

VHA Providers Do Not Always Adhere to Required Opioid Safety Risk Mitigation Strategies and Guideline Recommendations for Prescribing Opioids in a Safe Manner

VHA Providers at Selected Medical Facilities Do Not Consistently Follow Opioid Risk Mitigation Strategies

Our review of selected VHA medical facilities shows that providers do not always follow three key opioid risk mitigation strategies, two of which are required under VHA policy. Specifically, increasing the use of urine drug screening is an explicit goal of the OSI, and providers should generally ensure that an annual urine drug screening has been conducted.

VHA policy requires providers to 1) query state PDMPs at least annually when prescribing opioids to determine if the veteran has obtained opioid medications or other controlled substances from a non-VA provider and 2) obtain written informed consent from patients about the risks of initiating long-term opioid therapy.

These strategies are intended to help ensure that patients at VHA medical facilities are safely prescribed opioid medications. Overall, based on our review of 103 veterans at five selected facilities, we found that 75 percent of the veterans in our sample had an annual urine screening, 26 percent had their names queried in a PDMP, and 70 percent provided informed consent.[39]

Provider Adherence to Three Veterans Health Administration (VHA) Opioid Risk Mitigation Strategies at Five Selected Medical Facilities, March 2016 through March 2017

Increasing the use of urine drug screening is an explicit goal of VHA's Opioid Safety Initiative (OSI), and providers should generally ensure that an annual urine drug screening has been conducted. VHA policy requires providers to (1) query state prescription drug monitoring programs (PDMP) at least annually when prescribing opioids to determine if the veteran has obtained opioid medications or other controlled substances from a non-VA provider, and (2) obtain written informed consent from patients about the risks of initiating long-term opioid therapy. However, our review of medical records for a random nongeneralizable selection of 103 veterans subject to these risk mitigation strategies found that

Of the 53 veterans who received long-term opioid therapy:[a]

- 32 veterans received an annual urine drug screening, which allows providers to monitor the types of medications in a veteran's system, including controlled and illicit substances;
- 13 veterans had their names queried annually in a state PDMP to see if they had received prescriptions for controlled substances, including opioids from non-VHA prescribers; and
- 41 veterans had provided informed consent indicating that they had been educated on the risks and benefits of opioid use.

[39] Our findings related to urine drug screening and informed consent at the five selected VHA medical facilities are consistent with VHA data for all of its medical facilities. For the period April 1, 2017 through June 31, 2017, VHA data show that nationwide about 87 percent of veterans on long-term opioid therapy received an annual urine drug screening. For the period January 1, 2017 through March 31, 2017, about 83 percent of veterans who were prescribed long-acting or chronic short-acting (excluding schedule IV and V) opioids provided informed consent. However, our results are not consistent with nationwide VHA data for the period April 1, 2017 through June 31, 2017 showing that about 63 percent of veterans for whom long-acting or chronic short-acting opioids were prescribed had their names queried in a PDMP. This inconsistency is partly due to the fact that VHA did not require providers to query the PDMP until October 2016, 7 months into our review of patients from March 2016 to March 2017.

Of the 25 veterans prescribed an opioid and benzodiazepine concurrently: • 17 veterans received an annual urine drug screening; • 8 veterans had an annual PDMP query; and • 22 veterans had provided informed consent. Of the 25 veterans with the highest risk of an adverse event, such as a suicide, overdose, fall, or accident, based on their Stratified Tool for Opioid Risk Mitigation (STORM) risk score:[b] • 24 veterans received an annual urine drug screening; • 5 veterans had an annual PDMP query; and • 11 veterans had provided informed consent.

Source: GAO analysis of veterans' medical records. | GAO-18-380.

[a]VHA defines long-term opioid therapy as a 90-day supply of opioid medication prescribed in a 6-month period.

[b]The Stratified Tool for Opioid Risk Management (STORM) is designed to help providers estimate veteran risk for an overdose or suicide-related event and provide suggested interventions to mitigate that risk. It provides 1-year and 3-year risk categories (i.e., low, medium, high, and very high) reflecting a patient's risk of an adverse event if opioids are prescribed, based on the veteran's individual medical history and characteristics. The 25 veterans we reviewed had "very high" risk categories for both the 1-year and 3-year estimates. For example, a patient with an 18 percent risk of a suicide- or overdose-related health care event or death in the next year would be categorized as "very high" risk by the tool.

We identified a number of factors that may have contributed to the inconsistent adherence to the three key opioid risk mitigation strategies at our selected VHA medical facilities. These factors may impede providers' ability to consistently follow these strategies for all applicable patients at these facilities. To the extent that these factors are present across other facilities, VHA's ability to ensure that all veterans are prescribed opioids in a safe and effective manner may be limited.

PDMP Access Issues

Officials at four of the five selected medical facilities faced PDMP access issues. Officials at two facilities told us that not all facility staff can access state PDMPs due to state laws and regulations that do not allow access to all types of providers, such as nurses and pharmacists.[40] Officials

[40] The VHA directive requiring that providers query PDMPs notes that the requirement is subject to limitations imposed by states, which can impact VHA providers' access to PDMP databases.

at one of these selected facilities explained that nurse practitioners in that state cannot access the state's PDMP, so they must rely on other providers to obtain information from the PDMP about their patients. In addition, in some states, only providers licensed in the state may access the state's PDMP. Because providers at VHA facilities may not be licensed in the state where the VHA facility is located but licensed in another state, these providers may be unable to access the state's PDMP. Officials at two selected facilities also described difficulties accessing PDMPs in neighboring states that are part of the catchment area for the facility and where the veteran may reside. The low rates of adherence we identified may also be attributed to the fact that VHA did not require providers to query the PDMP until October 2016, 7 months into our review of patients from March 2016 to March 2017.

CARA directed VA to ensure access by VHA providers to information on controlled substances prescribing through state PDMPs, including by seeking to enter into memoranda of understanding with states to allow shared access of such information between states and the VA. According to VHA officials, VHA Central Office has not taken steps to develop memoranda of understanding with states, nor has it developed any related guidance. Officials said this issue is likely being addressed by individual VISNs and medical facilities. In addition, VHA officials told us they have communicated with Members of Congress and the National Governors Association to address issues related to VHA provider access to the state PDMPs.[41]

Lack of Required Staff to Support Providers

We also found that not all of the selected medical facilities and their respective VISNs had filled required staff positions that can help ensure provider adherence to opioid risk mitigation strategies—specifically, academic detailers and pain champions.

---

[41] An assessment of legal challenges affecting VHA providers' access to state PDMPs was outside the scope of our review.

- At the time of our review, not all facilities had access to VISN academic detailing services, which, according to VHA, can help ensure that providers follow opioid risk mitigation strategies. While VHA officials said that most VISNs across VHA had implemented an academic detailing program as required by VHA policy, two of the five VISNs for the selected facilities in our review had not.[42] Nationally, as of March 2018, four VISNs had not implemented an academic detailing program. Additionally, 11 facilities across VHA had not received a visit from a detailer.
- At the time of our review, four of five selected facilities did not have a Pain Champion as required by VHA policy beginning in March 2015.[43] Pain champions are generally primary care providers knowledgeable about pain care who can serve as a resource for other primary care providers by promoting safe and effective pain care. According to VHA officials, pain champions play a critical role in opioid safety and can help providers remedy gaps in pain care management for individual patients, such as incomplete opioid risk mitigation strategies.

Lack of Clinical Opioid Safety Alerts

Another factor that may limit adherence to the opioid risk mitigation strategies is the fact that none of the selected facilities employ electronic reminders to help remind primary care nurses of strategies that have not been completed. Primary care nurses are typically responsible for ensuring adherence to these strategies, and VHA facilities often employ electronic

[42] VHA requires that all VISNs fully implement an academic detailing program by September 30, 2015, defined as having at least three full time equivalent detailers. According to VHA Central Office officials, some VISNs have not met this requirement due to limits on the number of full time equivalent positions at the VISN. See VHA Memorandum, *System-wide Implementation of Academic Detailing and Pain Program Champions* (Washington, D.C.: March 27, 2015).

[43] VHA policy requires each medical facility to maintain a 0.25-0.50 full-time equivalent pain champion serving in primary care. See VHA Memorandum, *System-wide Implementation of Academic Detailing and Pain Program Champions* (Washington, D.C.: March 27, 2015).

alerts to notify providers when certain tasks need to be completed, such as regular screenings for depression and traumatic brain injury. Although VHA facilities are not required to develop these alerts, according to some primary care nurses we interviewed, it would be helpful to receive a reminder when a veteran is due for a PDMP query, urine drug screening, or has not given long-term opioid use informed consent. According to the nurses, such an alert could be issued through the electronic medical record system.[44]

Limited Facility Monitoring

We found that facilities' monitoring of provider adherence to the opioid risk mitigation strategies was limited across the five selected facilities in our review, which could hinder identification of non-adherence to these strategies. Specifically, while we found that all five medical facilities and VISNs in our review have an active pain management committee, facility officials told us that three of five facility committees do not conduct regular medical record reviews, which VHA encourages under its pain management directive to improve pain management.[45] The directive states that facility pain management committees should monitor the pain management practices at their facility. For example, the pain management committee could monitor providers' care plans for individual veterans, which are to be documented in the veterans' medical records. These types of medical record reviews could help identify providers who are not adhering to VHA's opioid safety requirements.

---

[44] According to facility officials, one facility in our review has alerts to remind prescribers to order a urine drug screening or query the PDMP when ordering an opioid. However, these alerts are not visible to primary care nurses.

[45] VHA's Pain Management Directive provides policy and implementation procedures for the improvement of pain management consistent with the VHA National Pain Management Strategy and compliance with generally accepted pain management standards of care. See VHA Directive 2009-053, *Pain Management*, (Washington, D.C.; October 28, 2009).

Some VHA Providers Do Not Consistently Follow Clinical Practice Guideline Recommendations Related to Opioid Safety

Provider Adherence to Selected Clinical Practice Guideline Recommendations for Management of Opioid Therapy for Chronic Pain at Five Selected Veterans Health Administration (VHA) Medical Facilities, March 2016 through March 2017

Clinical practice guidelines provide evidence-based recommendations designed to assist in provider decision-making; however, they are not VHA requirements and variations in practice will occur based on provider discretion and the needs of individual patients. Our review of medical records for a random, nongeneralizable selection of 103 veterans subject to the recommendations found that

Of the 53 veterans who had been prescribed long-term opioids:[a]

- 11 veterans were prescribed a non-pharmacological therapy, such as yoga, or cognitive behavioral therapy;
- 13 veterans were prescribed naloxone, which is a highly effective intervention for reversing an overdose;
- 29 veterans had a maintenance follow-up visit at least once every 30-180 days for the duration of the veteran's opioid therapy; and

3 of 21 veterans who had a change in their opioid medication during the time of our review had a follow-up visit between 14 and 28 days following the change.

Of the 25 veterans prescribed a concurrent opioid and benzodiazepine:

- 6 veterans were prescribed a non-pharmacological therapy;
- 4 veterans were prescribed naloxone;
- 11 veterans had a maintenance follow-up visit; and
- 0 of 9 veterans who had a change in their opioid medication during the time of our review had a follow-up visit between 14 and 28 days following the medication change.

Of the 25 veterans with the highest risk of an adverse event, such as a suicide, overdose, fall, or opioid-induced respiratory depression, based on their Stratified Tool for Opioid Risk Mitigation (STORM) risk score:[b]

- 4 veterans were prescribed a non-pharmacological therapy;
- 7 veterans were prescribed naloxone;
- 16 veterans had a maintenance follow-up visit; and
- 5 of 17 veterans who had a change in their opioid medication during the time of our review had a follow-up visit between 14 and 28 days following the medication change.

Source: GAO analysis of veterans' medical records. | GAO-18-380.

[a]VHA defines long-term opioid therapy as a 90-day supply of opioid medication prescribed in a 6-month period.

[b]The Stratified Tool for Opioid Risk Mitigation (STORM) is designed to help providers estimate veteran risk for an overdose or suicide-related event and provide suggested interventions to mitigate that risk. It provides 1-year and 3-year risk categories (i.e., low, medium, high, and very high) reflecting a patient's risk of an adverse event if opioids are prescribed, based on the veteran's individual medical history and characteristics. The 25 veterans we reviewed had "very high" risk categories for both the 1-year and 3-year estimates. For example, a patient with an 18 percent risk of a suicide- or overdose-related health care event or death in the next year would be categorized as "very high" risk by the tool.

We also found that some VHA providers at selected facilities do not consistently follow selected clinical practice guideline recommendations related to opioid safety. Our findings are based on our review of a random selection of medical records for 103 veterans prescribed opioids between March 2016 and March 2017. These guidelines recommend, for example, that providers consider using non-pharmacological treatments, such as acupuncture and yoga, for chronic pain and prescribe naloxone, a potentially lifesaving drug, as warranted. The guidelines provide evidence-based recommendations designed to assist in provider decision-making; however, they are not VHA requirements and variations in practice will occur based on provider discretion and the needs of individual patients. Overall, we found that, 20 percent of veterans in our sample were prescribed a non-pharmacological therapy, 23 percent of the veterans were prescribed naloxone, 54 percent had appropriate maintenance follow-up visits with a provider while prescribed opioids, and 17 percent had appropriate follow-up visits with a provider after a change in their opioid prescription. There are a variety of reasons that VHA providers may not always follow clinical practice guideline recommendations. For example, the availability of these non-pharmacological therapies may be limited, according to officials at all five selected VHA medical facilities. Officials at some facilities noted that the availability of these therapies can be particularly challenging for facilities in rural areas.

VHA officials explained that the biggest barrier to providing naloxone is educating providers, so that they consistently consider prescribing naloxone for their patients receiving opioid therapy.[46] According to officials, an education course for providers on naloxone prescribing became available in December 2015, and naloxone education efforts are a key focus of academic detailing programs. According to VHA data, since fiscal year 2014, naloxone distribution has increased. Specifically, as of

[46] Additionally, primary care nurses at the facilities in our review said they had difficulty finding adequate time and clinic space to provide the necessary education on naloxone to veterans when it was prescribed. They also described technological challenges, such as trying to show veterans education videos with audible sound on computers, and a lack of wireless internet access for the devices used.

March 2018, the agency has dispensed almost 142,000 naloxone kits to veterans, an increase of about 58 percent since June 2017.

CONCLUSION

VHA is taking important steps under the OSI to help ensure that veterans receive safe care. For example, VHA has begun tracking and publicly reporting data on four key metrics related to opioid prescriptions, and these data show that opioid prescription rates have decreased since 2013. In addition, our review also found that VHA has made progress on most of its 2014 OSI goals. However, for two goals, VHA lacks documentation showing whether VISNs and medical facilities have completed required relevant actions, and in one case, VHA has not specified measurable outcomes, which makes it challenging to determine whether these goals have been accomplished. Without sufficient documentation and measurable outcomes, VHA cannot determine whether these OSI goals to help ensure safe and effective care for veterans prescribed opioids have been fully successful.

Our review also shows that VHA needs to do more to ensure that its providers are following three key opioid risk mitigation strategies when prescribing an opioid medication to a veteran: conducting an annual urine drug screening, querying a PDMP, and obtaining written informed consent from the veteran on the benefits and risks of using opioid medications.

VHA has several means at its disposal for improving adherence to these strategies—at a minimum it should ensure that each VISN has a fully staffed academic detailing program and that each facility has a designated primary care pain champion, as VHA policy requires. In addition to enforcing these requirements, VHA should direct its facilities to strengthen monitoring efforts to help ensure providers' adhere to the opioid risk mitigation strategies. These efforts include regular reviews of veterans' medical records and creating electronic alerts reminding providers when these risk mitigation strategies have not been completed. Academic detailers and pain champions would also help educate providers further about evidence-based clinical practice guideline recommendations, such as non-pharmacological alternatives to opioid therapy and prescribing naloxone. Without these efforts to improve adherence to key opioid risk mitigation strategies, VHA's ability to ensure that all veterans are prescribed opioids in a safe and effective manner may be limited.

RECOMMENDATIONS FOR EXECUTIVE ACTION

We are making the following five recommendations to VA:

- The Undersecretary for Health should ensure that Central Office, VISNs, and medical facilities document the actions they take towards achieving OSI goals. (Recommendation 1)
- The Undersecretary for Health should ensure that any OSI goals that have not been met have clearly defined, measurable outcomes, including milestones or numerical targets, as appropriate, and timeframes. (Recommendation 2)
- The Undersecretary for Health should track the use of the OTRR (or any subsequent tool) by providers prior to initiating opioid therapy. (Recommendation 3)
- The Undersecretary for Health should ensure that all VISNs have implemented an academic detailing program that supports all medical facilities in the VISN and that all VHA medical facilities have a designated primary care pain champion as required. (Recommendation 4)
- The Undersecretary for Health should require VHA medical facilities to take steps to ensure provider adherence to opioid risk mitigation strategies, including querying PDMPs, obtaining written informed consent, and conducting urine drug screening. For example, these steps could include creating alerts in the electronic medical record system to remind primary care teams when these actions should be completed or strengthening facility monitoring of providers. (Recommendation 5)

AGENCY COMMENTS

We provided a draft of this chapter to VA for comment. While VA was reviewing a draft of this chapter, it requested further specificity in recommendation two; as a result, we revised the recommendation to be clearer. In its written comments, which are reproduced in appendix II, VA concurred with our recommendations and provided technical comments, which we have incorporated as appropriate. In its comments, VA agreed that clarifying ongoing priorities and plans and filling in gaps in implementation will help facilitate progress in its opioid safety efforts. VA stated that it will establish a workgroup to review all OSI goals and ensure that the goals have clearly defined measurable outcomes and timelines, and that documentation requirements are established. VA also informed us that in March 2018 it published a notice requiring VHA clinicians to conduct and document a data-based risk review using one of VHA's clinical decision support tools for opioid management, such as STORM, prior to initiating opioid therapy. VA also stated that it will take actions to ensure that academic detailing programs are fully implemented and primary care pain champions are in place across the system. To improve its clinicians' adherence to opioid risk mitigation strategies, VA stated that it will establish a workgroup to review and develop methods for increasing adherence. VA expects to complete all these actions by April 2019 or earlier. We are sending copies of this chapter to the appropriate congressional committees, the Secretary of Veterans Affairs, the Undersecretary for Health, and other interested parties.

A. Nicole Clowers
Managing Director, Health Care

List of Committees

The Honorable Johnny Isakson
Chairman

The Honorable Jon Tester
Ranking Member
Committee on Veterans' Affairs
United States Senate

The Honorable John Boozman
Chairman

The Honorable Brian Schatz
Ranking Member
Subcommittee on Military Construction, Veterans' Affairs, and Related Agencies
Committee on Appropriations
United States Senate

The Honorable Phil Roe
Chairman

The Honorable Tim Walz
Ranking Member
Committee on Veterans' Affairs
House of Representatives

The Honorable John Carter
Chairman

The Honorable Debbie Wasserman Schultz
Ranking Member
Subcommittee on Military Construction, Veterans' Affairs, and Related Agencies
Committee on Appropriations
House of Representatives

APPENDIX I: KNOWN EFFORTS AND DATA RELATED TO THE VETERANS HEALTH ADMINISTRATION'S (VHA) OPIOID SAFETY INITIATIVE (OSI) 2014 GOALS, JULY 2013-DECEMBER 2017

Table A-1.

OSI goals	VHA-required action(s)	Description of known related efforts and data
(1) Educate opioid prescribers regarding the effective use of urine drug screening	Each Veteran Integrated Service Network (VISN) must establish a network-wide standardized education program by December 31, 2014	According to VHA training system data, 13 of 21 VISNs developed at least one education course addressing the use of urine drug screening from January 1, 2015 through April 29, 2017. Ten of the 13 VISNs developed at least one course by the deadline (December 31, 2014) as required. Further, 6 of the 13 VISNs had at least one course with 30 or fewer providers completing it. Because we found the VISN course assignment data unreliable, we could not determine the completion rates for these courses. However, we found that, in response to a 2015 White House memorandum that required all federal employee opioid prescribers to complete training on the appropriate prescribing of opioids (which included discussion of urine drug screening) by April 15, 2017, of 20,231 prescribers who were identified and assigned the course, 19,242 completed it, for a completion rate of about 95 percent, according to VHA data from January 1, 2015 through April 29, 2017.
(2) Increase the use of urine drug screening	Urine drug screening targets based on previous urine drug screening rates for all VHA facilities must be reached by 2nd quarter, fiscal year 2015 (March 31, 2015)	According to VHA data, 151 of 157 facilities met or exceeded their urine drug screening target by the deadline (March 31, 2015) as required. In addition, VHA OSI metric data also show that there has been a 47 percentage point increase nationally in the percentage of patients on long-term opioid therapy who received a urine drug screen from the 4th quarter of fiscal year 2013 to the 1st quarter of fiscal year 2018. The increase in the percentage of patients receiving a urine drug screening was driven more by a reduction in the total number of patients on long-term opioid therapy rather than an increase in the number of patients receiving the screening.

Table A-1. (Continued)

OSI goals	VHA-required action(s)	Description of known related efforts and data
(3) Facilitate the use of prescription drug monitoring program (PDMP) databases, which contain patient-level information on prescriptions received for controlled substances	Each VISN must certify by 2nd quarter, fiscal year 2015 (March 31, 2015), that all facilities have a program consisting of PDMP training and/or education materials for providers	VHA Central Office lacks certifications from all VISNs that programs were established. Although officials at the five VISNs in our review told us they had supported training efforts on the use of PDMPs, only one VISN in our review provided documentation that it had established a program by the deadline (March 31, 2015) as required. However, in October 2016, VHA issued a directive requiring providers to query state PDMPs for patients prescribed opioids and also issued guidance on how PDMPs should be accessed and how these efforts should be documented in VA's electronic health record system. In addition, according to VHA officials, querying the PDMP was added to the 2015 White House-required opioid safety training, as described earlier. According to VHA data, there has been a 22 percent increase in the querying of PDMPs by providers from 4th quarter, fiscal year 2016 to 3rd quarter, fiscal year 2017.
(4) Establish safe and effective VISN tapering programs for veterans using opioids and benzodiazepines	VISNs must develop local tapering protocols and plans to resource the implementation of those tapering protocols	VHA Central Office lacks documentation from all VISNs regarding VISN-specific protocols and implementation plans. Only one of the five VISNs in our review provided documentation regarding a VISN-specific protocol relating to patients on opioids and benzodiazepines, which was developed in 2013. Four of the five VISNs did not provide documentation of a VISN-specific protocol or implementation plans.[a] However, VHA officials told us that they addressed this goal by issuing national tapering guidance including a provider reference guide in 2014, an opioid taper decision tool in 2016, and the VA/DOD clinical practice guideline in 2017. VHA officials said that the issuance of this guidance made the VISN-required action irrelevant. In addition, VHA OSI metric data show that there has been a 6.6 percentage point decrease nationally in the percentage of patients dispensed an opioid and benzodiazepine from the fourth quarter of fiscal year 2013 to the first quarter of fiscal year 2018.
(5) Develop tools to identify patients at a higher risk for adverse events while using opioids	An opioid risk stratification toolkit must be developed; opioid safety education guides must be updated annually	In 2016, VHA released its opioid risk stratification toolkit in the form of an opioid safety monitoring tool called the Stratification Tool for Opioid Risk Mitigation.[b] In addition, VHA updated its pain management opioid safety education guide and quick reference guide for providers in July 2017.

OSI goals	VHA-required action(s)	Description of known related efforts and data
(6) Improve prescribing practices around long-acting opioid formulations	VISNs must develop local tapering protocols and plans to resource the implementation of those tapering protocols	VHA Central Office lacks documentation from all VISNs regarding VISN-specific protocols and implementation plans. Only one of the five VISNs in our review provided documentation regarding a VISN-specific protocol relating to patients on opioids and benzodiazepines, which was developed in 2013. Four of the five VISNs did not provide documentation of a VISN-specific protocol or implementation plans.[a] As earlier described, VHA officials said that issuance of guidance nationally made the VISN-required action irrelevant. In addition, according to VHA data, the percentage of patients who were prescribed long-acting opioids by providers nationally has decreased by about 1 percentage point from quarter 3, fiscal year 2014 to quarter 3, fiscal year 2017, representing a decrease of about 44,000 patients prescribed long-acting opioids and an accompanying increase of about 223,000 patients who used VHA care in the last four quarters
(7) Review treatment plans for veterans on high doses of opioids[c]	Each VISN must certify that the treatment of all patients with a daily dose of greater than 200 morphine milligram equivalents has been reviewed by 2nd quarter, fiscal year 2015 (March 31, 2015)	VHA Central Office lacks certifications from all VISNs that reviews were conducted. Although officials at the five VISNs in our review told us they had completed these reviews, only one VISN provided us with documentation to conclude that its facilities completed their review. However, VHA OSI metric data show that there has been a 2.1 percentage point decrease nationally in the percentage of patients dispensed greater than or equal to 100 morphine milligram equivalents per day from the fourth quarter of fiscal year 2013 to the first quarter of fiscal year 2018.
(8) Offer complementary and alternative medicine modalities for chronic pain at all medical facilities	Each facility must provide evidence that at least two evidence-based behavioral/psychological treatments or approved complementary or alternative modalities can be provided by 2nd quarter, fiscal year 2015 (March 31, 2015)	According to VHA 2nd quarter, fiscal year 2015 data, all VHA medical facilities located in the United States provided at least one psychosocial service and at least one complementary and integrative health service.[d] However, VHA officials indicated that due to the nature of the data, they cannot verify that all psychosocial services provided at that time were evidence-based and that not all complementary and integrative health services provided had a strong evidence base.

Table A-1. (Continued)

OSI goals	VHA-required action(s)	Description of known related efforts and data
(9) Develop new models of mental health and primary care collaboration to manage the prescribing of opioids and benzodiazepines in patients with chronic pain	Identification of strong practices that can be operationalized across VHA by 3rd quarter, fiscal year 2015 (June 30, 2015); a request for proposal to be released to the field to establish model interdisciplinary teams and strategies for management and tapering of medications at three VHA medical facilities	In February 2016, VHA began a pilot to implement a model of care known as the Collaborative Chronic Care Model into existing Behavioral Health Interdisciplinary Program teams at nine VHA medical facilities. According to a VHA document, the pilot will provide facilitation support to enhance existing Behavioral Health Interdisciplinary Program teams by incorporating evidence-based Collaborative Care Model elements, which can include a care manager to proactively monitor care and progress as well as other tools intended to improve communication between primary care and specialty care. In fiscal year 2017, efforts were expanded to 30 additional VHA medical facilities. According to one VHA official, the pilot is expected to be completed no earlier than August 2019.

Source: VHA, GAO. | GAO-18-380.

Notes: OSI goals and required actions were issued via memorandum by VHA Central Office in December 2014. This table is not intended to be an exhaustive description of all of VHA's efforts related to its OSI goals.

VISNs are regional networks that manage the VHA medical facilities located in their area. In October 2015, VHA began to implement a realignment of its VISN boundaries which resulted in the number of its VISNs decreasing from 21 to 18.

[a]One VISN provided evidence of one VHA medical facility's tapering recommendations for patients on opioids and benzodiazepines.

[b]This tool helps providers identify patients who are at a higher risk of adverse events when using opioids depending on their clinical profile.

[c]Patients on high doses of opioids are at greater risk for adverse events. According to the Centers for Disease Control, providers should avoid or carefully justify opioid prescriptions delivering a daily dose of greater than or equal to 90 morphine milligram equivalents.

[d]Based on information we obtained from VHA relative to this goal, "psychosocial" services refer to "behavioral/psychological" treatments, and "integrated health" is a term that may be used to refer to "complementary and alternative" modalities. According to a VHA official, the VHA facility in Manila, the Philippines did not offer at least one psychosocial service and at least one integrative health service for this time period.

APPENDIX II: COMMENTS FROM THE DEPARTMENT OF VETERANS AFFAIRS

DEPARTMENT OF VETERANS AFFAIRS
WASHINGTON DC 20420

May 14, 2018

Ms. A. Nicole Clowers
Managing Director
Health Care
U.S. Government Accountability Office
441 G Street, NW
Washington, DC 20548

Dear Ms. Clowers:

The Department of Veterans Affairs (VA) has reviewed the Government Accountability Office's (GAO) draft report, ***"VA HEALTH CARE: Progress Made Towards Improving Opioid Safety but Further Efforts to Assess Progress and Reduce Risk Are Needed"*** (GAO-18-380).

The enclosure provides general and technical comments, and sets forth the actions to be taken to address the GAO draft report recommendations.

VA appreciates the opportunity to comment on your draft report.

Sincerely,

Peter M. O'Rourke
Chief of Staff

Department of Veterans Affairs (VA) Comments to
Government Accountability Office (GAO) Draft Report
"VA HEALTH CARE: Progress Made Towards Improving Opioid Safety but Further Efforts to Assess Progress and Reduce Risk Are Needed"
(GAO-18-380)

General Comments:

Thank you for the recognition of our innovation and progress. We agree that clarifying ongoing priorities and plans and filling in gaps in implementation will help facilitate progress in our continued Opioid Safety efforts. Our action plan describes how we plan to move forward on the recommendations.

Recommendation 1: The Undersecretary for Health should direct Central Office, VISNs, and medical facilities to document the actions they take towards achieving OSI goals.

VA Comment: Concur. The Department of Veterans Affairs (VA) agrees that continued actions and follow-up are important for tracking progress towards best clinical practices in opioid prescribing. The Veterans Health Administration (VHA) Office of Specialty Care will collaborate with the Office of Mental Health and Suicide Prevention to establish a workgroup to review all new Opioid Safety Initiative (OSI) goals; establish the expected metrics; timelines; and documentation requirements. The status is in process with a target completion date of April 2019.

<u>Recommendation 2</u>: The Undersecretary for Health should ensure that any OSI goals that have not been met or any new OSI goals that are developed in the future have clearly defined, measurable outcomes, including milestones or numerical targets, as appropriate, and timeframes.

<u>VA Comment</u>: Concur. VA agrees that continued actions and follow-up are important for tracking progress towards best clinical practices in opioid prescribing. VHA Office of Specialty Care will collaborate with the Office of Mental Health Suicide Prevention, within the established workgroup, to review and evaluate unmet goals that remain pertinent and will ensure all identified and pertinent unmet OSI goals are clearly defined and include measurable outcomes, milestones/metrics and timelines. The status is in process with a target completion date of April 2019.

<u>Recommendation 3</u>: The Undersecretary for Health should track the use of the OTRR (or any subsequent tool) by providers prior to initiating opioid therapy.

<u>VA Comment</u>: Concur. On March 8, 2018, VHA published VHA Notice 2018-08, *Conduct of Data-Based Case Reviews of Patients with Opioid-Related Risk Factors*. This notice requires VA clinicians to conduct and document a data-based risk review using one of VHA's clinical decision support tools for opioid management prior to initiating opioid therapy. The Notice established policy on implementation of OSI case reviews and provides instructions concerning the documentation of OSI case reviews within the medical record for patients with an opioid prescription identified as very high risk. VA's Stratification Tool for Opioid Risk Mitigation (STORM) has been adapted to facilitate this practice. Utilization of the standard progress note title will allow tracking of conduct and documentation of this practice. Pharmacy Benefits Management (PBM) Services, the Office of Specialty Care Services/Pain Management, in collaboration with Program Evaluation and Resource Center within the Office of Mental Health and Suicide Prevention, will host upcoming trainings on the utilization of the STORM tool within future months. The status is in process with a target completion date of July 2018.

<u>Recommendation 4</u>: The Undersecretary for Health should ensure that all VISNs have implemented an academic detailing program that supports all medical facilities in the VISN and that all VHA medical facilities have a designated primary care pain champion as required.

<u>VA Comment</u>: Concur. In regard to the implementation of Academic Detailing, the Office of the Assistant Deputy Under Secretary for Health for Clinical Operations (ADUSH C/O), with support from PBM Services, will issue a mandatory response for action via electronic mail, i.e., "tasker", on behalf of the Deputy Under Secretary for Health for Operations and Management (DUSHOM) to noncompliant Veterans Integrated Service Networks (VISN) no later than June 2018. The tasker will require the implementation of Academic Detailing programs as outlined in the March 2015, Office of Interim Under Secretary for Health memorandum. To ensure visibility and clarity, a copy of the March 2015, Memorandum will be sent with the tasker as an attachment. Additionally, the issued tasker will officially rescind any previously granted exemption waivers. Each VISN will be required to provide the Office of the DUSHOM and PBM with an attestation memorandum signed by the VISN Director with: 1) an anticipated implementation timeline; and 2) complete implementation of Academic Detailing within their respective VISN.

In relation to the designation of primary care pain champion, the Office of Specialty Care Services/Pain Management, in collaboration with the Office of Primary Care Operations (OPC), will assess VA medical facilities (VAMC) to ensure each VAMC has a designated primary care pain champion. Each VISN will be required to provide OPC with an attestation memorandum signed by the VISN Director. The status is in process with a target completion date of April 2019.

<u>Recommendation 5</u>: The Undersecretary for Health should require VHA medical facilities to take steps to ensure provider adherence to opioid risk mitigation strategies, including querying PDMPs and obtaining written informed consent (as required under VHA policy) and conducting urine drug screening, the increase of which is an OSI goal. For example, these steps could include creating alerts in the electronic medical record to remind primary care teams when these actions should be completed or strengthening facility monitoring of providers.

<u>VA Comment</u>: Concur. The Offices of Primary Care and Mental Health and Suicide Prevention, in collaboration with the National Center for Ethics in Health Care, will develop a workgroup to review and establish requirements concerning opioid mitigation

strategies to include educational materials, informed consent, urine drug screenings, decision-making tools, documentation, and the potential utilization of a national clinical reminder. The status is in process with a target completion date of April 2019.

INDEX

D

E

L

M

N

O

U

V

W